Stories on Disability Through Our Voices

This book integrates the discipline of disability studies with the lived experiences of women with visible disabilities. It seeks to foreground the silenced voices of Korean and Korean American women with visible physical disabilities in South Korea and the United States. Drawing upon the work of scholars in disability studies, largely drawn from disability studies in education and feminist disability studies, it challenges readers to (re)consider their own misconceptions and assumptions about disability and reconceptualize their understanding of diversity. A special distinction of this book is that the author, as a woman with visible disabilities, can connect to other women with visible disabilities in unique ways as they share similar experiences as well as their own unique stories through the process of in-depth interviews. Starting with a recollection of her own experience of living with a disability, it then moves to the lived experiences of four other women with disabilities. This unique way of storytelling conveys the important message that living with disability is not a one-time linear process from initial diagnosis to acceptance and overcoming, but a dynamic, evolving, and ongoing meaning-making journey. It will be of interest to all scholars and students of disability studies, Asian studies, women's studies, and sociology more broadly.

Yoon Joo Lee is Associate Professor in the Department of Childhood, Bilingual and Special Education, Brooklyn College, City University of New York, USA. She is the co-author of *Inclusion in the Early Childhood Classroom: What Makes a Difference?* New York, NY: Teachers College Press.

Autocritical Disability Studies

Series Editor
David Bolt
Liverpool Hope University, UK

This new book series represents both a contribution to, and a departure from, the academic field of critical disability studies. According to some concerns about that field, disability is the start but never the finish, there is insufficient engagement with the ethical and political issues faced by disabled people, and the work is too insensitive to individual experiences. Such concerns are addressed boldly in the new series via a formal coupling of critical disability studies with the research method of autoethnography.

The qualitative method of autoethnography acknowledges a researcher's individual experience in the most explicit of ways, from the very start of the process to the finished product that reaches publication. Whereas most traditional research methods claim, or at least aspire to, objectivity, autoethnography owns its subjectivity as paramount. This being so, when academic authors/editors have direct or at least intimate individual experience of disability, the subjectivity of their books can predicate a shift in typology from critical disability studies to what the new series terms autocritical disability studies.

In encouraging textual and theoretical work, the series also introduces autocritical discourse analysis and autocritical disability theory to formalise the ethical and epistemological importance of disability experience in many aspects of critical studies. The key point about the books sought for the series, then, is precisely that the individual experience of disability is recognised and positioned as both start and finish.

The book series editor, Professor David Bolt, encourages expressions of interest from potential monograph authors and volume editors.

Advertising Disability
Ella Houston

Stories on Disability Through Our Voices
Born This Way
Yoon Joo Lee

For a full list of titles in this series, please visit: https://www.routledge.com/Autocritical-Disability-Studies/book-series/ASHSERADS

Stories on Disability Through Our Voices

Born This Way

Yoon Joo Lee

Routledge
Taylor & Francis Group
LONDON AND NEW YORK

First published 2025
by Routledge
4 Park Square, Milton Park, Abingdon, Oxon OX14 4RN

and by Routledge
605 Third Avenue, New York, NY 10158

Routledge is an imprint of the Taylor & Francis Group, an informa business

ISBN: 978-1-032-74093-5 (hbk)
ISBN: 978-1-041-00310-6 (pbk)
ISBN: 978-1-003-60917-9 (ebk)

DOI: 10.4324/9781003609179

Typeset in Sabon
by Apex CoVantage, LLC

For Product Safety Concerns and Information please contact our EU representative: GPSR@taylorandfrancis.com
Taylor & Francis Verlag GmbH, Kaufingerstraße 24, 80331 München, Germany.

This book is dedicated to four remarkable women who shared their lives with honesty, grace, and humor. Your voices, your stories, and your reflections are the heart of this book, reshaping our understanding of what it means to live with disabilities with perseverance and strength, while navigating a world still learning to fully understand and embrace your diverse experiences. This book celebrates your unwavering determination and resilience. Thank you for sharing your narratives of hope, identity, and advocacy that continue to break barriers.

Contents

Figures

Acknowledgments

Writing this book has been a deeply rewarding and meaningful experience. I am deeply grateful to the four courageous women who shared their stories with such generosity and honesty. It has been an honor to celebrate their triumphs and accomplishments. Their ongoing efforts to live with purpose and aspiration encourage me to pursue my own life with the same determination.

I extend my sincere thanks to Claire Jarvis and the editorial team at Routledge for recognizing the potential of this project and guiding the review and publishing process with efficiency and care. Your unwavering support and encouragement made my first experience of writing a book as a sole author both smooth and positive.

This book would not have been possible without the support of many. In the early stages of writing, Dr. Hye Jun Park and Dr. David J. Connor graciously read my initial drafts and offered invaluable insights, guidance, and wisdom. I was also fortunate to receive the Wolfe Faculty Fellowship from Ethye R. Wolfe Institute for the Humanities at Brooklyn College, City University of New York, which provided me the rare opportunity to take a semester off from teaching and devote myself fully to this book. I am deeply thankful to Annie Yi for her editorial assistance – her help was instrumental in bringing this book to completion. I would like to thank Hye Min and Young Eun for their help with interview transcripts.

I am especially grateful to my family, friends, and colleagues, who have been a constant source of support and encouragement throughout this journey. I am blessed with a wonderful network of support and friendships that span different phases of my life. My heartfelt thanks go to my parents, my brother, and his family, for their love, encouragement, and unwavering belief in me. To my best friend, Joy – thank you for accepting me fully as who I am and never allowing me to use my disability as an excuse, no matter the challenge.

A central message of this book is the importance of recognizing the multiple identities of individuals with disabilities. As I reflect on my own life as a woman with a disability, I am reminded again of the profound significance of my identity as a Christian. Through this book, I hope to give glory to God.

It is my hope that this book serves as a modest catalyst for amplifying the voices of women with disabilities and bringing about positive change in their lives, helping to improve access and opportunities for them in the future.

Preface

My connection to this book goes beyond mere academic interest and is deeply grounded in both my personal and professional experiences. As a Korean American woman born with cerebral palsy, my lived experience is marked by multiple social identities. The main focus of my research has been education, specifically, social inclusion of children with disabilities and the successes and challenges of mothers raising children with disabilities. As I conducted more interviews with the parents of children with disabilities, I began to notice how my position as a person with physical disabilities, along with my personal experiences with cultural change, schooling, and disability, influenced the way I validated and interpreted participants' stories (Lee et al., 2015). Through these experiences, I have realized I am uniquely positioned to study the lived experiences of individuals with disabilities and disseminate their stories to a wider audience. This book evolved from my previous research and is more interdisciplinary, going beyond the field of education and addressing culture, gender, race, and disability.

I was born with mild cerebral palsy in South Korea. My disability clearly affects my walking, some of my fine motor skills, and my speech. I am not in a wheelchair and do not need assistive technology or equipment to function in my daily routine. However, my disability is visible enough that in any situation, my physical appearance stands out. Sometimes I have to repeat what I am saying when talking to strangers. I do not perceive myself as different from other nondisabled people just because I was born with cerebral palsy. I never had an experience with a "normal" body, so my physical disability is part of my everyday experience – I am just a person with disabilities, and I feel normal.

In this book, I intentionally use the term "encounter" to illustrate how my experiences of being disabled do not originate from inherent factors within myself or fixed deficits in my body. Through various social experiences, I face situations in which my way of being is deemed deficient or demeaned by others. When reflecting on my experience as a person with disabilities, I often think about how I have encountered stigmatization and how my cognitive and intellectual abilities have often been underestimated because of the visible nature of my disability. In this sense, I encounter "disability" in different social contexts. My story not only informs readers about the lived experience of disability but is also intertwined with the stories of other similarly positioned women to amplify that knowledge. This book begins with an account of my own disability experience to give readers a sense of who I am and my relevant encounters with disability.

My first significant encounter with my own disability

For the entire six years of elementary school, I attended a hospital-affiliated rehabilitation center, a special education school for children with physical disabilities and orthopedic impairments. I remember these years as happy times and do not recall any distinct encounters with my disability. When I was about to graduate from elementary school, I believe my mother recognized I had the potential to follow along in the general education curriculum. At that time, my parents' hope for me was to attend a four-year college. My mother believed that if I continued in special education schools, the teachers in these schools would set lower academic expectations for me. When she talked about sending me to a mainstream middle school, I was very anxious and did not want to face a world where I would be visibly different from others. I still remember how difficult it was to be the only student with disabilities in a huge public school. Back then, most students with disabilities attended segregated special education schools. Only a few were mainstreamed into public schools, and they had no formal support.

My first year in middle school was painfully challenging because, amidst the 2,500 teenage girls, it was the first time in my life that I clearly stood out. I can undoubtedly say this was the first time I really encountered my disability, realizing my body was different, not like anybody else's. That year, it was difficult for my peers to see me as who I was beyond the disability. My most vivid and painful memory is watching my peers looking at me as if they had never before seen a person with disabilities. When our homeroom teacher assigned a girl to sit next to me, she put her head down on the desk and began to cry. She didn't tell me directly why she was crying, but later that afternoon, I found that she cried because she thought my disability was contagious and that she would "catch" the disability from me. The homeroom teacher had to ask another student who was more tolerant to sit next to me. As I reflect back on that year, I realize how my homeroom teacher often intervened to make sure I would be taken care of and that someone from the class was "watching" me. Especially during field trips, she would tell the class president or vice president to take care of me, but those peers were not necessarily the group I hung out with. In retrospect, the teacher assumed that I didn't have any friends, so she assigned me a student. The teacher thought about caring and helping from a perspective based on certain assumptions about my (in)ability to make friends on my own. Even though I understood her good intentions, I resented them because I felt she had assumed I was someone who needed help. I thought to myself, "Do I not have a say in this?"

Because of my physical disability, I was initially perceived as helpless and not capable of doing many things. In middle school, I had to justify my presence in the mainstream setting with how well I performed academically and had to continuously convince teachers and other students that I could do well on tests. This might be because educational achievement is highly regarded in Korea. My mother was very supportive and determined to advocate on my behalf. At the beginning of every school year, she arranged for conferences with the homeroom teacher and the teachers who taught the other subjects so she could explain to them that my physical disability did not affect my cognitive or mental capacities.

My seventh-grade homeroom teacher was not happy when I was placed in her class and let me know about it indirectly. It was not because she was worried that I might be disruptive and present challenging behaviors. She was concerned that my grades might lower the class average and her reputation as a teacher might be undermined as a result. It took two months for her to realize that I was not the one bringing down the average test score of her class. When my grades showed that I was capable of following the general education curriculum, the perceptions of teachers and peers began to change. If I did well on a test, this teacher would show my report card to rebuke and pressure fellow classmates to do better. Teachers also commented to the class, "If she can get this score, you should be able to do so." I did not like that type of attention because I didn't want to stand out. Still, my academic performance became the standard that others used to judge me. I felt a constant need to prove to others that my physical disability did not mean I was slow.

A big transition: understanding other identifiers beyond disability

I grew up in a two-parent household with one younger brother. My father was the breadwinner of the family, and my mother was a full-time stay-at-home mom raising two children. My father worked at a large corporation in South Korea and was assigned to work in one of the company's overseas offices in Africa. After six years of working there and living apart from his family, he was given an opportunity to voice his preference for his next assignment. It might have been preferable and advantageous for him to transfer back to the main office in Korea, but after serious conversations with my mother, he submitted a request to be assigned to one of the offices in the United States. The company honored his request and assigned him to its satellite office in Texas. That is how I came to the United States as a teenager with my family. My parents made this big decision and sacrifice because it was my parents' priority to educate me in the United States so I could have more opportunities and access to education and employment.

It was very shocking and scary to start high school in a new country where I didn't speak a word of English. I felt like this was a bigger challenge than my initial experience of transitioning into mainstream middle school. During my high school years, I didn't think much about how my intellectual and cognitive abilities were underestimated because of the visible nature of my physical disability. When comparing my experiences in middle school in Korea and high school in the United States, I realize that in the United States, I was not as concerned with the need to prove my worth to others through my grades. Academic performance was not the standard by which students evaluated each other, but in Korea, it was the key to being accepted. Since Asian Americans are often held up as an example of the model minority, others did not see it as a big deal when I received good grades in math even though I was a student with disabilities. Getting good grades was not the way to integrate and be accepted into the school community. As I adjusted to the United States, I became more aware of my racial and cultural identities and, as a non-native English speaker, was more concerned with the language barrier than my disability identity. In class, I was afraid to raise my hand to speak, not because of my articulation issue related to my disability but my awkward English and heavy accent. From time to time, I was brave enough to speak up during math class because I just had to speak numbers in short phrases, but I didn't say a word in my English and U.S. history classes. Reflecting back on my experience of transitioning to life in the United States, I became more cognizant of how disability is a multivariant construct that is experienced intersectionally.

A lifelong journey of understanding intersectional identities in a disabled body: a Korean woman in New York

Sting wrote the song "Englishman in New York" after he was inspired by the famous eccentric Quentin Crisp, who jokingly remarked that he was waiting to receive his naturalization papers so that he could commit a crime and not be deported. This song resonated in my mind as I reflected on my experience as an international student living in the United States who wanted to seek permanent residence. I came to New York City to study in a graduate program in early childhood special education. I completed all the requirements for a master's degree, including full-time student teaching in a self-contained preschool classroom for children with physical impairments in a hospital-affiliated setting. During student teaching, I was often concerned about my physical limitations while working with children with physical disabilities. I was not able to move the children from their wheelchairs to special chairs during the instructional time. But this concern did not stop my desire and determination to become a special education teacher because I realized I could deal with this challenge by getting help from other professionals in the classroom. When I was about to complete the master's degree, I realized another significant factor affected my career path. Because I was an international student with a student (F-1) visa, I was not eligible for a New York State teaching license even after I completed all the requirements including the state certification tests, and this limited my choice to work as a special education teacher. At that time, only those with permanent residency (a Green Card) or U.S. citizenship were eligible to receive an initial teaching certificate in the state of New York. This was the first time I faced barriers that prevented me from accessing opportunities. It had nothing to do with my disability.

Since I was not able to go into full-time teaching, my choice was to either go back to Korea or continue my studies in a doctorate program because I could only stay in the United States with a student visa. I knew how access to full-time employment was still limited for people with disabilities in Korea. Therefore, I decided to stay by continuing my studies. Fortunately, after completing the doctorate degree, I went into full-time teaching at a college, and it was easier to get a Green Card through this job.

I am very grateful and feel privileged to have studied in the United States. I was given access to a wide range of opportunities, and America has definitely opened doors to more opportunities for individuals with disabilities. I have often wondered if I would have been able to achieve all that I have if I had lived in Korea. However, as a woman of color whose first language is not English, I have experienced marginalization because of multiple aspects of my identity, including disability. Many times, these intersecting identities have significantly impacted my life. In particular, during the summer of 2021, Asian hate crimes increased significantly, and like all my Korean American friends, I felt uncomfortable with riding the subway and walking on the streets of New York City. During my previous 20 years of living in the New York metropolitan area, I had always been comfortable and had no problem using public transportation despite my physical disability. When the number of the Asian hate crimes increased, I became very cautious and concerned because the presence of race was more clearly visible on me because my manner of walking stood out in the crowd. On the busy streets of the city, I did not feel safe as an Asian woman with a visible disability. By sharing about this incident, I highlight the importance of understanding the intersection of other identifiers such as gender, race, and culture, instead of focusing on only disability.

From living in two countries, South Korea and the United States, I have seen how different social and cultural contexts impacted the formation of my disability identity. I am an emergent bilingual whose first language is Korean and who had the experience of being caught in a space where I needed to negotiate between two cultures. Thus, my lived experience is marked with multiple social identities. This book begins with some of my own stories with the hope that my journey can be a starting point for readers to understand how I am uniquely positioned to present the stories of other women with visible disabilities. My positionality is key to the conceptualization of this book, recruitment of its participants, theoretical framework, and analytical lens. By presenting stories of four women with disabilities along with my story, I hope to portray the dynamic and multidimensional aspects of living with disabilities as a lifelong journey, as well as individuals' multiple identities beyond disability. Overall, it is a book not just about disability, but about life.

Reference

Lee, Y.-J., Park, H. J., & Recchia, S. L. (2015). Embracing each other and growing together: Redefining the meaning of caregiving a child with disabilities. *Journal of Child and Family Studies*, *24*(12), 3662–3675. https://doi.org/10.1007/s10826-015-0175-x

1 Introduction

The untapped power of first-person narratives: breaking the silence of Korean women with physical disabilities

In our own voices: authentic storytelling beyond supercrip narratives

"Born This Way," by famous pop artist Lady Gaga, is a song about celebrating individual differences, freedom, and feminism. The message of this song resonates deeply in the core of individuals with disabilities who understand disability as human variation and disability identity as a way of being in the world. Garland-Thomson (2014) shared that she is often asked, "What's wrong with you?" regarding her physical impairment and asymmetrical hands, and her personal narrative response is "I was born this way." She explained that this response, instead of reflecting her experience of discrimination in the world, where disability is primarily understood as something gone terribly wrong, reflects the formation of her disability identity, "disabled knowing," and her intention to establish a claim to inclusion and access to resources.

The experiences of people with disabilities are often told from the perspectives of their families and the professionals who work with them. The voices of disabled people themselves are not prevalent (Sherry, 2016). Hence, this book, *Stories on Disability Through Our Voices: Born This Way*, explores the lived experiences of Korean and Korean American women with visible disabilities in South Korea and the United States. Foregrounding their voices, this book attests to the significant impact of narratives of disability and situates the meanings of their experiences within cultural and social contexts by addressing the following key questions:

1. How do the lived experiences of Korean and Korean American women with disabilities in South Korea and the United States shape their subjective lives and their perspectives on the future as well as their views on education, work, and employment?
2. How do they articulate their disability identity as they talk about their lives?
3. How is their disability identity uniquely situated within their cultural contexts?
4. How do they negotiate self-perception related to disability identity and others' perceptions of disability?

DOI: 10.4324/9781003609179-1

In this book, women with disabilities are agentic in producing counternarratives (Bamberg, 2004), which assign new meaning to lived experiences, in contrast to master narratives (Andrew, 2004), which are dominant constructions assumed to be the normative experience. Counternarratives offer perspectives that challenge social expectations and widespread beliefs and problematize dominant viewpoints on human experiences (Lalvani & Polvere, 2013; Solórzano & Yosso, 2002). Another important purpose of counternarratives is to bring into scholarship the lives and experiences of "those people whose experiences are not often told (i.e., those on the margins of society)" (Solórzano & Yosso, 2002, p. 34). In studies that seek to provide those individuals the chance to speak and be heard, subjectivity is recognized and valued, meaning that an emic perspective is gained with emphasis placed on people and their subjective lived experiences (Moriña, 2020). Therefore, this book focuses on how people talk about their own disabilities. They acknowledge their differences, celebrate moments of achievement, and go through the ordinary ups and downs of life. At the same time, they engage in a constant process of problem-solving to deal with challenges and difficulties associated with their disabilities. Presentations of their lives include extraordinary moments of success in the midst of barriers, as well as ordinary and mundane aspects.

Sheldon (2017) discussed the importance of a research format that allows the disabled person to play the role of a primary researcher in disability research. By following the tradition of storytelling, this book attests to the untapped power of this type of research. It is an important addition to the body of work that "centers the wisdom of disabled people" (Wong, 2020, p. xx). In the field of disability studies, storytelling is an important tool for presenting the unique perspectives of individuals with disabilities (Smith-Chandler & Swart, 2014) and privileging their voices (Rogers-Shaw, 2022). Several books (e.g., Connor, 2008; Wong, 2020) have focused on these alternative voices, portraying their lived experiences. In Connor (2008), the experiences of young people of color (Black and Latino) with invisible disabilities were delivered in their own words, in the form of poetry and drawings. In Wong (2020), a collection of stories about disabled people illustrated multidimensional aspects of their lives. This book offers a unique contribution by presenting the voices of Korean and Korean American women with disabilities, who are virtually absent from educational research, as they talk about school, work, and other lived experiences.

Success stories of individuals with disabilities, known as supercrip narratives (Berger, 2008; Schalk, 2016), tend to focus on courage, dedication, and hard work, and convey the message that these individuals can defy the odds and accomplish the impossible. These stories are likely to be perpetuated to inspire others but can lead to the unrealistic expectation that one can achieve anything if one only tries hard enough (Berger, 2008). The supercrip is a potentially damaging stereotype of disability that must be challenged (Schalk, 2016). By elevating the "ordinary" lived experiences of women with physical disabilities as worthy of study, this book serves to deconstruct prevalent notions of "overcoming" disability, defying narratives of the supercrip. The intention of this book is not to inspire others through fairytales focusing on the success of individuals with disabilities or to elicit empathy for all the obstacles they have experienced. Instead of merely addressing disability-related issues, the book aims to present the experience of living with disabilities as an ongoing journey characterized by dynamic and multidimensional aspects. It explores the various identities of individuals beyond disability within the framework of disability studies. In essence, this book delves into the broader spectrum of human diversity that touches all of our lives.

Theoretical framework: perspectives on disability

Born This Way is consciously grounded in an interdisciplinary and critical approach largely drawn from feminist disability studies, critical disability studies, and disability studies in education. Disability studies, the overarching field that provides the foundational principles for these subdisciplines, challenges traditional medical models of disability and embraces a social model for understanding disability. This social model views disability not as a deficit but as a natural human variation. Rather than an individual or medicalized phenomenon, disability is a phenomenon that occurs within specific cultures and contexts through social, cultural, and historical interpretation (Connor et al., 2012). Disability is characterized as socially created through an association between impairments and discriminatory behaviors and attitudes in society (Hutchinson et al., 2018).

Disability studies in education (DSE) specifically examines how disability is understood and experienced in educational contexts through research topics involving inclusive classrooms, educational policies (e.g., Ruppar et al., 2022), and the experiences of disabled students and parents (e.g., Daelman et al., 2022). DSE scholars have challenged the foundation of traditional special education, which emphasizes disability as an intrinsic personal dysfunction (Anastasiou & Kauffman, 2011; Slee et al., 2021). Connor (2020) explained how this deficit-based thinking manifests in demarcations along lines of race, social class, and gender that categorize students into certain disability labels, and this has led to disproportionality in inclusive classrooms. As resistance against the oppression of students with disabilities in and through education, DSE emphasizes the centering of disabled people in generating new forms of research and practice that challenge ableist traditions in special education (Slee et al., 2021). DSE has "invigorated explorations around the broad area of disability and education in numerous ways, a welcome contrast to the stilted, barely moving pace of developments in theory, research, and practice within the field of special education" (Connor, 2020, p. 31). In this book, the stories of four women with disabilities address several issues of inclusion, access, and belonging in their educational experiences in special education schools as well as mainstream settings.

Critical disability studies (DisCrit) takes disability studies a step further by incorporating critical theories (e.g., critical race theory, feminist theory) to analyze power structures, systemic inequalities, and social justice issues that contribute to the marginalization of people with disabilities. Within this framework, it is understood that disability is often experienced as both a biomedical problem of body and mind, and a social and political one based on factors such as social exclusion, poor social welfare, and inaccessible public infrastructure (Flynn, 2021). Annamma et al. (2018) developed seven tenets for the DisCrit framework, which many researchers have applied to challenge traditional ways of thinking about disabilities. For example, Ocasio-Stoutenburg (2021), who recounts her journey as a mother of a Black male child with a visible disability, applied the third tenet of DisCrit to illustrate how (dis)ability labeling is socially constructed and has manifested in a focus on deficits rather than a holistic view of individuals as people with feelings, opinions, and rights. The second tenet is closely intertwined with this book and emphasizes the value of acknowledging multidimensional identities and troubling singular notions of identity. In the context of Korean society, the intersection of gender, disability, and class has positioned women with disabilities in historically marginalized positions, as evidenced by the lives of the four women in this book, whose experiences have been shaped by various intersecting factors beyond disability.

Feminist disability studies influences many aspects of this project. Feminist disability studies focuses on intersections between feminism and disability and recognizes culture as a key site where disabled women have been historically misrepresented (Houston, 2019). Disabled women are doubly disadvantaged and in parallel ways because of cultural expectations, received attitudes, and social institutions (Garland-Thomson, 2001). Kafer (2013) incorporated a political/relational model of disability into her research, stating, "Disability is experienced in and through relationships; it does not occur in isolation" (p. 8). Therefore, the major goal of this field is to explore how gender and disability intertwine to create exclusionary, oppressive systems for disabled women, for the purposes of countering prejudice, understanding disability as a political issue, and building a shared community (Simplican, 2017). A recent example of such exploration is Houston (2019), which showed how feminist disability studies can be applied to critique the exploitation of women with mobility impairments in 21st-century advertising.

Rosemarie Garland-Thomson (2005, 2011), a prominent scholar in feminist disability studies, employed a method of sharing disabled women's narratives to dismantle sexist and ableist assumptions and explore how disabled women may reclaim identities denied them in popular culture. She emphasized the importance of exploring how gender interlocks with race, ethnicity, sexuality, and class systems. Garland-Thomson (2006, 2009) also described staring as a process that establishes a social relationship between the starer and the staree. Staring can be "a social act that stigmatizes by designating people whose bodies or behaviors cannot be readily absorbed into the visual status quo" (2009, p. 44). This act of staring resonates with the experiences of Korean women with physical disabilities in this project because the visible nature of their disabilities often makes their physical presence stand out as abnormal and unusual in many social situations in Korean culture.

As there is a dynamic interplay between the subdisciplines of disability studies, this book seeks to draw on insights from multiple areas to develop a more comprehensive understanding of disability and its intersections with education, critical theory, and gender. The relationships between these fields demonstrate the interdisciplinary nature of disability studies and its capacity to address complex and interconnected aspects of human experience (Connor, 2020). Many scholars in disability studies have addressed the political, cultural, and sociological significance of disability/impairment identities (Hutchinson et al., 2018; Mpofu & Harley, 2006; Sherry, 2016; Watson, 2002). Disability identity is defined as "a cultural-developmental phenomenon by which an individual with a disability incorporates into his or her self-definition his or her own disability-related difference and regards that difference as a resource for participation in normative activities of his or her society" (Mpofu & Harley, 2006, p. 16). The notion of a disabled identity can be imposed on individuals as their defining identity even though it is only a part of who they are (Hutchinson et al., 2018). However, disability is a multivariant construct that is experienced intersectionally (Friedensen & Kimball, 2017). Therefore, it is critical to present lived experiences within a frame of intersectionality, taking into account the intersections between factors such as race, class, gender, sexuality, place, and age, to examine cultural constructions of disability as a whole (Sherry, 2016).

Garland-Thomson (2014) explained that disability identity is formed when a characteristic of a person manifests as atypical or abnormal in social environments through interactions with others. For example, an individual's physical impairment is recognized as a disability through appearance while someone with autistic spectrum disorder is identified as disabled through their functioning in social contexts. Disability identity can be affected by prevailing societal norms and values associated with impairments that can further foster discriminatory and stereotypical behaviors (Hutchinson et al., 2018). In this book, I explore the extent to which such sociocultural factors have influenced the participating women's disability identities by analyzing their narratives of lived experiences.

Disability identity is not the same as acceptance of disability (Mpofu & Harley, 2006). Even when individuals may be accepting of their disability, they may consider it a deficit that they wish they did not have. On the contrary, disability identity is developed when a person self-identifies with their disability and sees it as a positive experience that enriches their life. To explore disability identity at a deeper, more authentic level and the messy nature of lived experiences, it is important to consider how disability relates to all identity markers, such as class, gender, and race (Hirschmann, 2013), instead of defining people solely based on the nature of their impairment. It is problematic to ascribe disabled people to a single fixed and preordained group according to disability (Watson, 2002). Loja et al. (2013) also emphasized the importance of intersections among multiple social identities such as gender, disability, race, class, and sexuality in shaping one's experiences and opportunities. Several studies (Banks, 2018; Guerrero-Arias et al., 2020; Slater et al., 2018) have examined how the disability experience is woven throughout individuals' multiple identities. Banks (2018) uncovered characteristics of the interaction of disability and race through a case study of an African American male with cerebral palsy, while Guerrero-Arias et al. (2020) and Slater et al. (2018) explored the intersectionality of disability, race, and gender through portraits of women with disabilities from minority backgrounds. *Born This Way* also addresses the social construction of disability identity with an intersectional approach. Additionally, it captures the changing nature of disability identity across life stages. Norton (2000) explained the defining characteristics of social identity within a poststructuralist framework; identity is multiple, decentered, and even contradictory as we go through different experiences in the social world, and it changes over time as we pass through life stages. We "constantly reconfigure ourselves through multiple identities, and time space and relationality are all important in identity formation" (Watson, 2002, p. 511).

Disciplines under the overarching field of disability studies place high value on the use of storytelling to privilege the voices of individuals with disabilities. In addition to qualitative interviewing techniques, many researchers in DisCrit embrace the fourth tenet, which emphasizes the importance of privileging the individuals themselves, who are not traditionally acknowledged but marginalized as research participants (Annamma et al., 2018). Scholars in feminist disability studies, such as Garland-Thomson and Kafer, also use life writing to advance theoretical understanding of disability (Simplican, 2017). Disability life writing has been described by Johnson and McRuer (2014) as writing that aims at "knowing and unknowing disability, making and unmaking disability epistemologies, and the importance of challenging subjects who confidently 'know' about 'disability'" (p. 130), as though it could be a thoroughly comprehended piece of knowledge. Many DSE scholars have incorporated the method of storytelling into their research to foreground disabled individuals and their families and present various aspects of disability experiences, such as inclusion, isolation, and access (Connor & Berman, 2019; Rogers-Shaw, 2022; Valente & Danforth, 2016). For example, through her own story as a disabled woman living through the COVID-19 pandemic and the stories of her students with disabilities, Rogers-Shaw (2022) illustrated the power of storytelling, focusing on a more holistic view of disability for the purpose of moving away from labels. *Born This Way* adheres to the central belief in disability studies that recognizes all women have multiple identities and diverse life histories and that their voices, standpoints, and experiences need to be validated. The stories in this book are organized to develop a direct testimony of the lived realities of individuals whose experiences are marked with multiple social identifiers.

Cultural and social backdrop

South Korea is one of the few countries where nationality and ethnicity coincide. An ideology of sameness dominates many aspects of Korean society, from attitudes toward domestic and international politics (Grinker, 2007) to kinship, adoption, and marriage (Kim, 2007). Homogeneity, solidarity, oneness, and conformity with the norm are consciously and subconsciously ingrained in the lives of individuals and families. Therefore, Koreans are extremely concerned with *siseon*, how one is judged and perceived by others (Kim, 2012). For example, Korean mothers of children with disabilities may be reluctant to accept diagnoses of their children because they are concerned about others seeing them as standing out from their peers (Grinker & Cho, 2013). Portrayed as a disruption of the culture of conformity, disability presents a social problem that reflects long-held prejudices about those who do not fit in (Woo, 2012). In Korea, persons with disabilities tend to be viewed as ones who at best should be pitied or treated as objects of charitable goodwill, so they often experience prejudice and discrimination. Employment opportunities remain limited despite the mandatory disability employment system (Disability Rights Support Division, 2019). Microaggressions can be caused by a lack of understanding of the characteristics of disability or sensitivity to the damage caused by conflicts of interests (Park, 2017). Disabled women in particular are economically vulnerable due to high unemployment rates and low-income levels compared to disabled men (Kim, 2010).

Similar cultural values and mindsets significantly influence life for Korean Americans in the United States. Several studies on Korean families of children with disabilities in Korea and the United States have shown the similarity in their cultural mindsets (Kwon et al., 2010; Lee & Park, 2016; Lee et al., 2015; Park & Chung, 2015). In Kwon et al. (2010) and Lee and Park (2016), stories from immigrant Korean mothers in the United States illustrate their high sense of responsibility regarding their children's education and how strongly they prioritized the facilitation of their children's academic success, a phenomenon called *gyoyukyeol*, or education fever. However, despite a number of studies on the experiences of their families and the professionals who work with them, a lack of research presents the lived experiences of individuals with disabilities themselves in Korea and the United States. Therefore, this book brings unique perspectives to the body of literature on disability experiences as it presents the stories of disabled women in their own words, by their own accounts. Through these stories, I hope to present a holistic view of disability, although not a universal one.

Born This Way explores how cultural expectations and assumptions impact disability identity. Cultural perspectives affect people's perceptions, which can distort and hinder the way they see people with disabilities (Kim, 2012). When addressing the cultural construction of disability in Korea, the perspective that is presented most is that of the families of children with disabilities (e.g., Grinker & Cho, 2013; Kim, 2012). There are a small number of studies that incorporate the voices of individuals with disabilities. For example, in a study addressing the complex combination of women's issues and disability issues in Korea, Kim (2010) exhibited the voices of leaders in disabled women's advocacy organizations in the country. Even though these leaders had lived experiences as women with disabilities who had worked hard to develop professional competencies, the findings focused on successes and challenges related to the operation of the advocacy agencies. The powerful stories of how these women stepped into leadership positions that affected the lives of other people with disabilities were not explored.

The voices of Korean and Korean American women with disabilities have been silenced and are virtually absent from the body of research about disability experiences. In the United States, Asian Americans are seen as the model minority, an exemplar of a racial minority that has achieved academic, economic, and social success through hard work and good ethics (Park et al., 2021; Yoo et al., 2010). This stereotype oversimplifies the diverse experiences within the Asian American community and can perpetuate harmful stereotypes. Even the positive aspects of the model minority stereotype have made a certain population particularly vulnerable (Park et al., 2021). For Asian Americans, disability is especially invisible and thereby unintelligible within the discourse of the model minority myth (Chang, 2018). Chang (2018) commented, "The obfuscation of disability is not only caused by the model minority myth but is also fundamental to the myth's creation" (p. 243). Therefore, there is a significant need to provide a compelling and necessary means of critiquing stereotypes such as the model minority myth through the integration of disability studies into Asian American studies (Chew, 2019). *Born This Way* serves this purpose.

Description of the research

Utilizing autoethnography

A special distinction of this book is that I, as a woman with visible disabilities, was able to connect to other women with visible disabilities in unique ways as we shared similar experiences as well as our own unique stories through the process of in-depth interviews. Even though I strongly believe in the impact of my own identities, I also acknowledge that having a similar background did not automatically afford me an emic (insider) perspective on the lives of participants with the same disability or the same racial background. I constantly engaged in the process of deconstructing my own disability and examining social context to move away from superficial understandings of disability (Sheldon, 2017). The sociological method of autoethnography aims to reject hierarchies between the researcher and research participant and embrace an explicit goal of transformation (O'Dea, 2018). By integrating my own disability experiences into this book, I illustrate one of the affordances of autoethnography, which is "not simply to document personal experience [or] evoke emotional resonance with the reader [but rather] to gain insight into some broader set of social phenomena" (Anderson, 2006, p. 387). Autoethnography involves inquiry that is both highly personal and scholarly to offer a unique perspective on an issue (Jones, 2020). An autoethnographic account documents and shares a personal story (Lourens, 2018).

Autoethnography may be defined as a highly personalized qualitative research methodology. It is not only a research methodology but also a way of life (Bochner, 2020). Researchers using autoethnography incorporate their personal experiences to describe, question, and reflect on lived experiences and interactions with others in sociocultural contexts (Adams, 2012; Adams et al., 2017; Smith, 2017). They see themselves as a part of what they study and often write stories about the research process and their experiences (Ellis & Adams, 2020). Autoethnography not only permits but encourages a focus on self-understanding. "Epiphanies," remembered moments perceived to have significantly impacted the trajectory of a person's life (Ellis et al., 2010), are included to illustrate relevant issues. Researchers using autoethnography focus on the outward social and cultural aspects of their own experiences, after which they look inward, examining how one is influenced by cultural interpretations (Adams, 2012; Congdon, 2014; Ellis & Bochner, 2000). Thus, autoethnography is both a process and a product (Ellis et al., 2010). Autoethnographers incorporate mainly reflective, dyadic interviews, exploring deeply the personal experience that brought them to the topic and what they learned about themselves and their emotional responses in the course of interviewing (Ellis & Berger, 2001). Personal experience is used to complement interview data, emphasizing the researcher's thoughts, feelings, and subjective positions as well as the participants' stories (Ellis & Adams, 2020).

Autoethnography has been used to explore lived experiences of disability and describe individual stories of past, present, and prospective future experiences of living with disabilities (e.g., Jones, 2020; McKinney, 2018; O'Dea, 2018). It has been utilized to bring insights into social perceptions, the formation of disability identity, everyday experiences, educational experiences, discrimination, and advocacy and empowerment. Some autoethnographic studies focus on the role of parents as advocates for their children with disabilities. They include narratives of empowerment, activism, and the challenges faced in advocating for disability rights and inclusivity. Ocasio-Stoutenburg (2021) chose autoethnography to sketch her journey toward advocacy as a Black woman and mother of a son with Down syndrome as well as a parent advocate for other children with disabilities from marginalized backgrounds. As a methodological choice, autoethnography breaks the traditional bounds of academic writing, weaving in storytelling with scholarship and blurring researcher – writer boundaries.

Scholars with disabilities have shared their stories in autoethnographic format to suggest the importance of learning something new about the subtle continua of disability identity (Jones, 2020) and the need for a shift in social perceptions of people living with disabilities (O'Dea, 2018). Lourens (2021a, 2021b) wrote about her journey in academia from doctoral student to university lecturer through the method of autoethnography. As she reflected back on difficult portions of her life as an individual with visual impairments, she was able to unravel unconscious experiences, thoughts, and memories by looking inward to thoughts and emotions and outward to external realities. Kasnitz (2020) also explored her biopolitical positioning as disabled through analysis of her dialogue with colleagues and students in a university setting. Their works are good examples of the therapeutic power of autoethnography beyond the purposes of advocacy and empowerment because they illustrate how this research can be used to disclose hidden details of private life and highlight emotional experience (Bochner, 2012; Lourens, 2021a).

In this autoethnographic research, I am an insider, and this enables living with disabilities to be portrayed as a lifelong journey with dynamic and multidimensional aspects. The participating individuals' multiple identities beyond disability are highlighted instead of being turned into "inspirational porn." I start this book with my own story and share my experiences throughout. As the other women's stories are told in each chapter, I discuss similar themes that emerged during the interview process and how I have reinterpreted my own experiences. My story has been significantly affected by their stories, and I describe how they have contributed to my thinking and feelings about issues related to lived experiences. Bochner (2000) suggested that autoethnographies contain "abundant" and "concrete" details, "not only facts but also feelings" (p. 270) and Ellis (2009) pointed out the importance of exploring what stories of the past mean now. Not only do my experiences inform readers about the lived experience of disability, but my story is also intertwined with the stories of other similarly positioned women to amplify that knowledge. Their stories are presented along with my own as a woman with visible disabilities.

Data collection method

My method of data collection included a series of three in-depth interviews with four participants. These interviews were conducted via Zoom at times that were convenient for each individual. The model of phenomenological interviewing was used to explore the meaning of the participants' experiences in the context of their lives (Seidman, 2019). During the first interview, which focused on life history, participants were asked to tell as much as possible about themselves, including their childhood, schooling experiences, and families, up to the present. The purpose of the second interview was to capture in detail their professional experiences and their talk about their careers. In the third interview, participants were asked to reflect on how their lived experiences affected their present and future. All the interviews were conducted in Korean and recorded, and then transcribed in Korean and translated into English. The participants, who were given the option to use pseudonyms, were provided with the interview transcripts in Korean for a member check and were allowed to review their completed chapter. Follow-up Zoom interviews were conducted to discuss their final reflections. They shared their thoughts on the portrayal of their story, highlighting intriguing sections and unexpected inclusions. Moreover, they were encouraged to talk about the impact of their participation in this book and reflect on how the whole process, from interviews to the review of the written chapter, influenced their lives.

The participant group was relatively small, as researching life histories involves in-depth study (Moriña, 2020). I interviewed four women with visible physical disabilities between 40 and 52 years of age. In terms of selection criteria, I incorporated the positive deviance approach, which focuses on "behaviors or conditions that overconform to normative expectations that are also positively evaluated" (Heckert & Heckert, 2004, p. 78). By learning from individuals who rise above cultural and social expectations and assumptions about women with disabilities, valuable knowledge can be gained about aspects of their lives and support networks, and how these factors can be used as powerful methods of change in the lives of other individuals with disabilities. I focus on physical disability in this book because I also have a physical disability and am particularly interested in attitudes toward the body. Three out of the four women have cerebral palsy, and one woman has Laing distal myopathy, a slowly progressing muscle disorder. All have undergraduate degrees, and three have master's degrees. Additionally, two of these women have earned doctorate degrees. All of them have established stable careers. Three live in Korea, while one lives in the United States. Although they share common experiences, the four women are not a homogeneous group and are very different as individuals.

The perspective of this book is unique because my identities help bridge the gap between researcher and participant, offering a point of connection and common experience. My "disabled identity" appeared to signal shared experiences. Finlay (2002) highlighted the profound impact that the personal identities of researchers have on the research process. Different markers of my identities significantly impacted my whole process, beginning with the desire to write down the stories of women with disabilities that resonate with my own background and experiences. I believe I was able to understand the gender, cultural, and socioeconomic issues that emerged from the participants' narratives; however, even though I strongly believe in the impact of my own identities, I also acknowledge that having a similar background does not automatically afford me an emic perspective on the lives of participants with the same disability or the same racial background. Reflexivity played an important role as I recruited the participants, interviewed them, and wrote their stories. Through this research process, I constantly engaged in the process of deconstructing my own disability and examining social context to move away from superficial understandings of disability (Sheldon, 2017). Throughout each chapter, I attend to my own identities (ethnicity, socioeconomic status

(SES), gender, age, disability). McDevitt (2021) articulated the process of becoming a reflective researcher as she interviewed immigrant teachers. Her work is a great example of research experience turning into something more meaningful as she shared feelings of marginalization with immigrant teachers. The same process is embedded throughout this book.

Overview of the book

Following this introductory chapter, the stories of the four women with visible disabilities are individually featured in Chapters 2–5. In creating each woman's story from the interview transcripts, I sought to preserve their wholeness and authenticity by weaving their words throughout the chapters. Each story is presented as a whole, without the interruption of scholarly interpretation. To establish consistency across the stories, each chapter is divided into the following three sections.

Encountering: "to come upon face to face"

Each woman's story starts with two encounters. First, I describe how I am connected to each woman in this project and how I recruited them. The second encounter refers to how each woman faced the realities of her own disability and how she related to early memories and anecdotes illustrating how the disability was experienced in and through relationships (Kafer, 2013). In addition, these stories show each woman's experience of prejudice and assumptions in Korean and/or American society.

Embracing: "accept or support willingly and enthusiastically"

In this section, the narratives focus on how each woman has embraced her own disability through negotiation and problem-solving in situations they have faced. This section is about embracing challenges and possibilities beyond the expectations of others as well as our own. Each woman talks about how her disability is embraced by significant people in her life and describes the process of being accepted and supported for who she is despite discrimination and marginalization at the larger societal level.

Intersection between her story and my story

During the interview process, I noticed that these women's stories resonated with my own experiences. As I listened to them, memories I had forgotten came back to mind. When I shared my experiences with them, their responses made me rethink and reflect on my past, and I was able to engage in a more in-depth analysis of my own experience of disability. At the end of each chapter, I share how interviewing these women made me reinterpret my experiences.

A unique issue emerged from each story

Each chapter ends with a brief discussion of a distinctive theme arising from the respective narrative. These themes are often specific to each woman's story, presenting insights that may not neatly align with preceding discussions. They include topics such as the intersectionality of disability with other aspects of identity or noteworthy perspectives introduced by individual women.

More specific descriptions of each chapter's contents are offered below.

Chapter 2 Hee-Yeon: reconnecting with a childhood friend striving to articulate the multivariant nature of disability identity

Hee-Yeon is a 47-year-old woman with cerebral palsy who works as an editor in a publishing company. She loves to read and invests her time and energy into ongoing professional development (e.g., studying Japanese with the hope of translating a Japanese book into Korean). Before she started working full-time at the publishing company, she worked for an advocacy group for women with disabilities in Korea and shared her disability experiences in short essays in the organization's newsletter. Hee-Yeon is a childhood friend with whom I went to a special education school for children with orthopedic impairments in Seoul, Korea, for six years.

Chapter 3 Jinju: living in the body of a disabled person with the perspective of a nondisabled individual

Jinju is a 40-year-old woman with Laing distal myopathy, the severest of the physical challenges experienced by the four women. She is a disability advocate and doctoral student whose major is in social welfare. It was fascinating to hear how she has lived with the perspective of a nondisabled individual at certain points in her life. Jinju attended only mainstream schools with nondisabled peers from elementary to high school. It was not until her college years that she found opportunities to socialize with other individuals with disabilities and study with them. She shared her process of discovering her own biases and assumptions toward other people with disabilities during college. Her Christian faith was also an important part of her narrative.

Chapter 4 Theresa: questioning moments of marginalization and moving beyond barriers

Theresa is a 40-year-old woman with cerebral palsy who lives and works in a city three hours from Seoul. She works as a disability advocate in a nonprofit organization and runs the local branch. She is also an athlete who competes in a wheelchair at the National Sports Festival for People with Disabilities. Theresa brings unique insights into the role of special education schools in Korea. She grew up in a rural area where inclusion with nondisabled peers was rarely implemented compared to schools in Seoul. From a very young age, she had wanted to go to school with her nondisabled peers but was denied by local schools. Because she was denied attendance in mainstream schools, she attended segregated special education settings from elementary to high school.

Chapter 5 Helen: reflecting on her experience in academia

Helen is a 52-year-old Korean American woman with cerebral palsy living in the United States and working as a professor who teaches special education classes at a university. She is fluent in both English and Korean. She came to the United States after high school and completed her undergraduate and graduate degrees at U.S. universities. Since completing her doctorate, she has been working as a full-time professor. She is married with two young adult children.

Chapter 6 "Life goes on": the continuous journey of living with a disabled body

This final chapter summarizes important themes that emerged from my analysis of the follow-up interviews with the individual participants. This chapter underscores the book's commitment to authentically portraying the participants' experiences, foregrounding their voices to the greatest extent possible. Additionally, common threads observed across all four narratives are explored. The purpose is not to generalize disability experiences but to discuss common issues to address the significant impact that social and cultural contexts have on the lives of individuals with disabilities.

Contribution to the field

Born This Way is a relevant and meaningful addition to the body of work that acknowledges the importance of insider accounts of disability to understand the embodied experience of disability (Garland-Thomson, 2005). This book offers a unique contribution by presenting the voices of Korean and Korean American women with disabilities and putting their lives and experiences at its center. The intersections of gender and other identities have shaped their experiences, including the intersection of disability and Asian culture. The contents of this book may be of great interest to those who want to see how disability studies and the method of storytelling can be incorporated to present and empower the voices of people with marginalized identities. My own disability experiences are integrated with the stories of the women to delve deeper into issues and highlight themes surrounding physical disability.

This book attempts to deconstruct existing stereotypes that depict people with disabilities as always passive and requiring help from others, and it seeks to describe how they become active agents who make positive changes and contributions in their lives and in the lives of those around them. This book is not about their stories but about *our* stories, and our views on disabilities are reflected in "how we use words and what stories we tell" (Rogers-Shaw, 2022, p. 8). These stories of women with disabilities will be accessible and compelling to those – family members, educators, advocates, policymakers – who are personally and professionally connected to individuals with disabilities. As different constituencies understand the perspectives of those with lifelong disability identities, they will be able to broaden their understanding of disability. These stories convey the important message that living with disability is not a one-time, linear process from diagnosis to acceptance to overcoming, but a dynamic, evolving, and ongoing meaning-making journey.

References

Adams, T. E. (2012). The joys of autoethnography. *Qualitative Communication Research*, *12*(1), 181–194. https://doi.org/10.1525/qcr.2012.1.2.181

Adams, T. E., Ellis, C., & Jones, S. H. (2017). Autoethnography. *The International Encyclopedia of Communication Research Methods*, 1–11. https://doi.org/10.1002/9781118901731.iecrm0011

Anastasiou, D., & Kauffman, J. M. (2011). A social constructionist approach to disability: Implications for special education. *Exceptional Children*, *77*(3), 367–384. https://doi.org/10.1177/001440291107700307

Anderson, L. (2006). Analytic autoethnography. *Journal of Contemporary Ethnography*, *35*(4), 373–395.

Andrews, M. (2004). Memories of mother: Counter-narratives of early maternal influence. In M. Bamberg & M. Andrews (Eds.), *Considering counter narratives* (pp. 7–26). Amsterdam: Benjamins.

Annamma, S. A., Ferri, B. A., & Connor, D. J. (2018). Disability critical race theory: Exploring the intersectional lineage, emergence, and potential futures of DisCrit in education. *Review of Research in Education*, *42*(1), 46–71. https://doi.org/10.3102/0091732X18759041

Bamberg, M. (2004). Considering counter narratives. In M. Bamberg & M. Andrews (Eds.), *Considering counter narratives* (pp. 351–371). Amsterdam: Benjamins.

Banks, J. (2018). Invisible man: Examining the intersectionality of disability, race, and gender in an urban community. *Disability & Society*, *33*, 894–908. https://doi.org/10.1080/09687599.2018.1456912

Berger, R. J. (2008). Disability and the dedicated wheelchair athlete: Beyond the "supercrip" critique. *Journal of Contemporary Ethnography*, *37*, 647–678.

Bochner, A. P. (2000). Criteria against ourselves. *Qualitative Inquiry*, *6*(2), 266–272. https://doi.org/10.1177/107780040000600209

Bochner, A. P. (2012). On first-person narrative scholarship: Autoethnography as acts of meaning. *Narrative Inquiry*, *22*(1), 155–164. https://doi.org/10.1075/ni.22.1.10boc

Bochner, A. P. (2020). Autoethnography as a way of life: Listening to tinnitus teach. *Journal of Autoethnography*, *1*(1), 81–92. https://doi.org/10.1525/joae.2020.1.1.81

Chang, Y. (2018). Asian American, disability and the model minority myth. In C. J. Schlund-Vials (Ed.), *Flashpoints for Asian American studies* (pp. 241–253). Fordham University Press.

Chew, K. (2019, February 25). Disability studies and Asian American literature. *Oxford Research Encyclopedia of Literature*. Retrieved 13 September 2024, from https://oxfordre.com/literature/view/10.1093/acrefore/9780190201098.001.0001/acrefore-9780190201098-e-912

Congdon, M. J. (2014). What's wrong with me? An autoethnographic investigation of the co-cultural communicative practices of living with Tourette syndrome during adolescence. *The Qualitative Report*, *19*, 1–25. https://doi.org/10.46743/2160-3715/2014.1411

Connor, D. J. (2008). *Urban narratives: Portraits in progress, life at the intersections of learning disability, race, and social class*. New York, NY: Peter Lang.

Connor, D. J. (2020). "I don't like to be told that I view a student with a deficit mindset": Why it matters that disability studies in education continues to grow. *Canadian Journal of Disability Studies*, *9*(5), 19–41. https://doi.org/10.15353/cjds.v9i5.689

Connor, D. J., & Berman, D. (2019). (Be)Longing: A family's desire for authentic inclusion. *International Journal of Inclusive Education*, *23*(9), 923–936. https://doi.org/10.1080/13603116.2019.1602361

Connor, D. J., Valle, J. W., & Hale, C. (2012). Forum guest editors' introduction: Disability studies in education "at work." *Review of Disability Studies: An International Journal*, *8*(3), 5–13.

Daelman, S., De Schauwer, E., & Van Hove, G. (2022). Connective collaboration around Alex – A constant searching around inclusive education. *Journal of Disability Studies in Education*, *3*(1), 29–56. https://doi.org/10.1163/25888803-bja10015

Disability Rights Support Division. (2019, April 30). The combined second and third periodic report under the convention on the rights of persons with disabilities. *Ministry of Health and Welfare*. http://www.mohw.go.kr/react/al/sal0301vw.jsp?PAR_MENU_ID=04&MENU_ID=0403&BOARD_ID=140&BOARD_FLAG=00&CONT_SEQ=349275

Ellis, C. (2009). *Revision: Autoethnographic reflections on life and work*. Walnut Creek, CA: Left Coast Press.

Ellis, C., & Adams, T. E. (2020). Practicing autoethnography and living the autoethnographic life. In P. Leavy (Ed.), *The Oxford handbook of qualitative research* (2nd ed., pp. 359–396). Oxford University Press.

Ellis, C., Adams, T. E., & Bochner, A. P. (2010). Autoethnography: An overview. *Forum: Qualitative Social Researcher*, *12*(1), https://doi.org/10.17169/fqs-12.1.1589

Ellis, C., & Berger, L. (2001). Their story/my story/our story. In J. F. Gubrium & J. A. Holstein (Eds.), *Handbook of interview research* (pp. 849–875). Thousand Oaks, CA: Sage.

Ellis, C., & Bochner, A. (2000). Autoethnography, personal narrative, reflexivity: Researcher as subject. In N. Lincoln & Y. Lincoln (Eds.), *The handbook of qualitative research* (2nd ed., pp. 733–768). Thousand Oaks, CA: Sage.

Finlay, L. (2002). "Outing" the researcher: The provenance, process and practice of reflexivity. *Qualitative Health Research*, *12*(4), 531–545. https://doi.org/10.1177/104973202129120052

Flynn, S. (2021). Corporeality and critical disability studies: Toward an informed epistemology of embodiment. *Disability & Society*, *36*(4), 636–655. http://dx.doi.org/10.1080/09687599.2020.1755237

Friedensen, R., & Kimball, E. (2017). Disability as identity: A critical examination of a multivalent construct. In J. Huisman & M. Tight (Eds.), *Theory and method in higher education research* (pp. 229–247). Emerald Publishing.

Garland-Thomson, R. (2001). *Reshaping, re-thinking, re-defining: Feminist disability studies*. Washington, DC: Center for Women Policy Studies.

Garland-Thomson, R. (2005). Feminist disability studies. *Signs*, *30*(2), 1557–1587. https://doi.org/10.1086/423352

Garland-Thomson, R. (2006). Ways of staring. *Journal of Visual Culture*, *5*(2), 173–192. https://doi.org/10.1177/1470412906066907

Garland-Thomson, R. (2009). *Staring: How we look*. Oxford University Press, Incorporated.

Garland-Thomson, R. (2011). Integrating disability, transforming feminist theory. In K. Hall (Ed.), *Feminist disability studies* (pp. 13–48). Bloomington, IN: Indiana University Press.

Garland-Thomson, R. (2014). The story of my work: How I became disabled. *Disability Studies Quarterly*, *34*(2). https://doi.org/10.18061/dsq.v34i2.4254

Grinker, R. R. (2007). *Unstrange minds: Remapping the world of autism*. Basic Books.

Grinker, R. R., & Cho, K. (2013). Border children: Interpreting autism spectrum disorder in South Korea. *Ethos*, *41*(1), 46–74. https://doi.org/10.1111/etho.12002

Guerrero-Arias, B., Agudelo-Orozco, A., & Pava-Ripoll, N. (2020). Intersectional identity chronotopes: Expanding the disability experience. *Disability & Society*, *35*(10), 1660–1681. http://dx.doi.org/10.1080/09687599.2020.1719041

Heckert, A., & Heckert, D. M. (2004). Using an integrated typology of deviance to expand Merton's anomie theory. *Criminal Justice Studies*, *17*(1), 75–90. http://dx.doi.org/10.1080/08884310420001679352

Hirschmann, N. (2013). Disability, feminism and intersectionality: A critical approach. *Radical Philosophy Review*, *16*(2), 649–662. https://doi.org/10.5840/radphilrev201316247

Houston, E. (2019). 'Risky' representation: The portrayal of women with mobility impairment in twenty-first-century advertising. *Disability & Society*, *34*(5), 704–725. http://dx.doi.org/10.1080/09687599.2019.1576505

Hutchinson, K., Roberts, C., & Daly, M. (2018). Identity, impairment and disablement: Exploring the social processes impacting identity change in adults living with acquired neurological impairments. *Disability & Society*, *33*(2), 175–196. https://doi.org/10.1080/09687599.2017.1392931

Johnson, M. L., & McRuer, R. (2014). Cripistemologies: Introduction. *Journal of Literary & Cultural Disability Studies*, *8*(2), 27–147.

Jones, P. (2020). On being a zebra: Negotiating a professional identity whilst coping with a rare and recurrent illness. *The Qualitative Report*, *25*(6), 1713–1720. https://doi.org/10.46743/2160-3715/2020.4295

Kafer, A. (2013). *Feminist, queer, crip*. Bloomington, IN: Indiana University Press.

Kasnitz, D. (2020). The politics of disability performativity: An autoethnography. *Current Anthropology*. *61*, S16–S25. https://doi.org/10.1086/705782

Kim, E. (2007). Our adoptee, our alien: Transnational adoptees as specters of foreignness and family in South Korea. *Anthropological Quarterly*, *80*(20), 497–531. https://doi.org/10.1353/anq.2007.0027

Kim, H. U. (2012). Autism across cultures: Rethinking autism. *Disability & Society*, *27*(4), 535–545. https://doi.org/10.1080/09687599.2012.659463

Kim, K. M. (2010). The accomplishments of disabled women's advocacy organizations and their future in Korea. *Disability & Society*, *25*(2), 219–230. https://doi.org/10.1080/09687590903537448

Kwon, K. Y., Suh, Y., Bang, Y. S., Jung, J., & Moon, S. (2010). The note of discord: Examining educational perspectives between teachers and Korean parents in the U.S. *Teaching and Teacher Education*, *26*, 497–506.

Lalvani, P., & Polvere, L. (2013). Historical perspectives on studying families of children with disabilities: A case for critical research. *Disability Studies Quarterly*, *33*(3). https://doi.org/10.18061/dsq.v33i3.3209

Lee, Y.-J., & Park, H. J. (2016). Becoming a parent of a child with special needs: Perspectives from Korean mothers living in the United States. *International Journal of Disability, Development and Education*, *63*(6), 593–607 https://doi.org/10.1080/1034912X.2016.1154139

Lee, Y.-J., Park, H. J., & Recchia, S. L. (2015). Embracing each other and growing together: Redefining the meaning of caregiving a child with disabilities. *Journal of Child and Family Studies*, *24*(12), 3662–3675. https://doi.org/10.1007/s10826-015-0175-x

Loja, E., Costa, M. E., Hughes, B., & Menezes, I. (2013). Disability, embodiment and ableism: Stories of resistance. *Disability & Society*, *28*(2), 190–203. https://doi.org/10.1080/09687599.2012.705057

Lourens, H. (2018). Driving in unheard silence: Disability and the politics of shutting up. *Journal of Health Psychology*, *23*(4), 567–576. https://doi.org/10.1177/1359105316643856

Lourens, H. (2021a). Giving voice to my body: Healing through narrating the disabled self. *Disability & Society*, *36*(6), 849–863. https://doi.org/10.1080/09687599.2020.1778445

Lourens, H. (2021b). Supercripping the academy: The difference narrative of a disabled academic. *Disability & Society*, *36*(8), 1205–1220. https://doi.org/10.1080/09687599.2020.1794798

McDevitt, S. E. (2021). "Don't be afraid": Exploring methodological relationships in (re)searching the experiences of immigrant teachers of color. *Multicultural Perspectives*, *23*(1), 40–47. https://doi.org/10.1080/15210960.2021.1877543

McKinney, E. M. (2018). Two's company, three's a crowd: Disabled people, their careers and their partners. *Disability & Society*, *33*(2), 272–284. https://doi.org/10.1080/09687599.2017.1399106

Moriña, A. (2020). Using life history with students with disabilities: Researching with, rather than researching on. *Educational Review*, *72*(6), 770–784. https://doi.org/10.1080/00131911.2018.1550054

Mpofu, E., & Harley, D. A. (2006). Racial and disability identity: Implications for the career counseling of African Americans with disabilities. *Rehabilitation Counseling Bulletin*, *50*(1), 14–23. https://doi.org/10.1177/00343552060500010301

Norton, B. (2000). *Identity and language learning: Gender, ethnicity and educational change*. Malaysia: British Library.

Ocasio-Stoutenburg, L. (2021). Becoming, belonging, and the fear of everything black: Autoethnography of a minority-mother-scholar-advocate and the movement toward justice. *Race Ethnicity and Education*, *24*(5), 607–622. https://doi.org/10.1080/13613324.2021.1918401

O'Dea, Z. (2018). The ayes have it! *The Qualitative Report*, *23*(10), 2313–2336. https://doi.org/10.46743/2160-3715/2018.2897

Park, H. J., & Chung, G. H. (2015). A multifaceted model of changes and adaptation among Korean mothers of children with disabilities. *Journal of Child and Family Studies*, *24*, 915–929. https://doi.org/10.1007/s10826-014-9902-y

Park, J. Y. (2017). Disability discrimination in South Korea: Routine and everyday aggressions toward disabled people. *Disability & Society*, *32*(6), 918–922. https://doi.org/10.1080/09687599.2017.1321223

Park, M., Choi, Y., Yoo, H. C., Yasui, M., & Takeuchi, D. (2021). Racial stereotypes and Asian American youth paradox. *Journal of Youth and Adolescence*, *50*(12), 2374–2393. https://doi.org/10.1007/s10964-021-01519-8

Rogers-Shaw, C. (2022). Disabled lives & pandemic lives: Stories of human precarity. *Occasional Paper Series*, *2022*(47). https://doi.org/10.58295/2375-3668.1435

Ruppar, A. L., Kurth, J. A., McCabe, K. M., Toews, S. G., McQueston, J. A., & Johnston, R. (2022). Present levels of academic achievement and functional performance: Unravelling the narratives. *Journal of Disability Studies in Education*, *3*(1), 4–28. https://doi.org/10.1163/25888803-bja10016

Schalk, S. (2016). Reevaluating the superscript. *Journal of Literary & Cultural Disability Studies*, *10*(1), 71–86. https://doi.org/10.3828/jlcds.2016.5

Seidman, I. (2019). *Interviewing as qualitative research: A guide for researchers in education and the social sciences* (5th ed.). Teachers College Press.

Sheldon, J. (2017). Problematizing reflexivity, validity, and disclosure: Research by people with disabilities about disability. *The Qualitative Report*, *22*(4), 984–1000. https://doi.org/10.46743/2160-3715/2017.2713

Sherry, M. (2016). A sociology of impairment. *Disability & Society*, *31*(6), 729–744. https://doi.org/10.1080/09687599.2016.1203290

Simplican, S. C. (2017). Feminist disability studies as methodology: Life-writing and the abled/disabled binary. *Feminist Review*, *115*, 46–60. https://doi.org/10.1057/s41305-017-0039-x

Slater, J., Agustsdottir, E., & Haraldsdottir, F. (2018). Becoming intelligible woman: Gender, disability and resistance at the border zone of youth. *Feminism and Psychology*, *28*, 408–426. https://doi.org/10.1177/0959353518769947

Slee, R., Corcoran, T., & Best, M. (2021). Disability studies in education – Building platforms to reclaim disability and recognise disablement. *Journal of Disability Studies in Education*, *1*(1–2), 3–13. https://doi.org/10.1163/25888803-00101002

Smith, B. (2017). *Narrative inquiry and autoethnography*. London: Routledge International Handbooks.

Smith-Chandler, N., & Swart, E (2014). In their own voices: Methodological considerations in narrative disability research. *Qualitative Health Research*, *24*(3), 420–430. https://doi.org/10.1177/1049732314523841

Solórzano, D. G., & Yosso, T. J. (2002). Critical race methodology: Counter-storytelling as an analytical framework for education research. *Qualitative Inquiry*, *8*(1), 23–44. https://doi.org/10.1177/107780040200800103

Valente, J. M., & Danforth, S. (2016). Disability studies in education: Storying our way to inclusion. *Occasional Paper Series*, *2016*(36). https://doi.org/10.58295/2375-3668.1158

Watson, N. (2002). Well, I know this is going to sound very strange to you, but I don't see myself as a disabled person: Identity and disability. *Disability & Society*, *17*(5), 509–527. https://doi.org/10.1080/09687590220148496

Wong, A. (2020). *Disability visibility: First-person narratives from the twenty-first century*. New York, NY: Vintage Books.

Woo, C. W. (2012). "Seeing another/seeing oneself": Nondisabled audiences' perspectives on disability in two South Korean films. "Oasis" (2002) and "Malaton" (2005) [Doctoral dissertation, Syracuse University].

Yoo, H. C., Burrola, K. S., & Steger, M. F. (2010). A preliminary report on a new measure: Internalization of the Model Minority Myth Measure (IM-4) and its psychological correlates among Asian American college students. *Journal of Counseling Psychology*, *57*(1), 114–127. https://doi.org/10.1037/a0017871

2 Hee-Yeon

Reconnecting with a childhood friend striving to articulate the multivariant nature of disability identity

> 한국 사회가 굉장히 사회적 약자에 대해 매우 살기가 안 좋잖니, 차별과 혐오는 여전히 나타나고 표면적으로 드러나고, 그래서 나는 왜 한국인 장애여성을 특히 강조를 했냐 하면, 한국에서의 장애여성은 그만큼 억압을 받고, 불평등하고, 어쩌면 한쪽으로 이렇게 빗겨 있는 존재. 안 보여야 할 존재.
>
> 한국에서 장애인으로 산다는 것? 나같이 어딘가 장애를 가지고 사는 건, 아무것도 보상이 없는 거야. 보상도 없고 아무것도 없는 . . . 바다에서 헤엄치고 있는 것과 똑같아. 언제 내가 헤엄을 멈추고 언제 죽게 될지 모른다는 것.
>
> [It's very challenging for the socially disadvantaged to live in Korean society. Discrimination and hatred rise to the surface. The reason why I emphasized that I identified as a Korean woman with a disability is, in Korea, women with disabilities experience more discrimination and rejection, almost to the point where they need to live undetected – invisible beings.
>
> What is it like to live as a disabled person in Korea? If you're living with disabilities like me, there's no reward for anything. No rewards, nothing . . . . It's like swimming in the ocean, in that I don't know when I'm going to stop swimming and when I'm going to drown.]
>
> – Hee-Yeon

Hee-Yeon is a 47-year-old woman with cerebral palsy. She works as an editor in a publishing company, editing and revising book manuscripts before final revisions. Occasionally, she is asked to translate manuscripts. The largest portion of her work is through one company, but since she works from home, she often takes freelance projects to supplement her income. She does a little bit of her own writing and is trying to publish her own book about her lived experience of disability. She can walk independently without a wheelchair or cane, but her speech/articulation issues are significant enough that it may be difficult for people to understand her speech when they hear her for the first time or if they are not used to her speech. Out of all the women who are represented in this book, Hee-Yeon had the most significant speech/articulation issues, and her speech was the most difficult to understand.

DOI: 10.4324/9781003609179-2

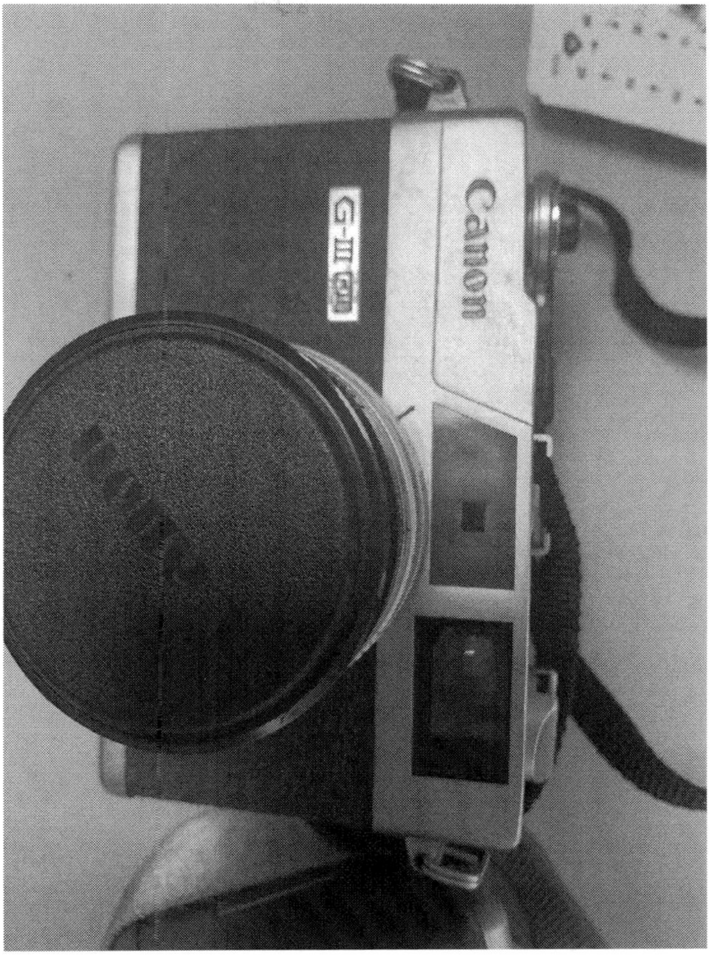

Figure 2.1 Hee-Yeon's camera: capturing meaningful moments

Hee-Yeon loves to read and invests her time and energy in ongoing professional development. For instance, she is studying Japanese with a private tutor with the hope of working on a book project that involves translating a Japanese book into Korean. Hee-Yeon also likes to travel, and one of her favorite hobbies is taking photographs when she visits different places. She submitted the following picture of a camera (Figure 2.1) and talked about the special meaning and contemplation behind her photograph:

> As I started taking more pictures, my eyes became open to perceiving things differently. A photo holds more than just a superficial visual image; it is a record of the thoughts, memories, and feelings of that moment. When

> I look at the photos later, I reflect on why I took this picture at that time, and it becomes a record of me. Even though I'm taking pictures of other people, these pictures are more like who I saw at that time, how I saw and felt about that person, and that showed up in the photo. I came to appreciate taking pictures of others as well as being in photos, since it becomes a way to cherish the moment. People assume that I am not capable of taking good photos because of the spasms in my hands due to my disability.

Contrary to assumptions people make, Hee-Yeon did not consider herself to be physically limited in handling a camera and taking pictures.

Before working full-time at the publishing company, Hee-Yeon worked as an outreach coordinator/researcher in an advocacy group for women with disabilities in Korea for about four years. Her responsibilities included creating materials such as flyers, pamphlets, and magazines and sharing her disability experiences in short essays in the organization's newsletter.

Hee-Yeon was born and raised in South Korea. She was the oldest child in a two-parent household and has a brother who is 12 years younger. After six years in a special education elementary school for children with orthopedic impairments, she transitioned to a mainstream setting for middle and high school. She did not pass the college entrance exam upon graduation from high school, so she attended a community college for a semester. She was not satisfied with her community college experience since it did not provide the educational experience she wanted. By the time she applied to university for a second time and retook the exam, there were legal mandates in Korea providing accommodations for students with disabilities in terms of college entrance exams. Thanks to this special admissions process, Hee-Yeon was able to enter one of the most prestigious universities in Korea. She wanted to major in Korean language and literature, but there were too many people with disabilities applying for that major. The special admissions process only assigned a certain number of students to specific majors, so she decided on sociology. She eventually majored in sociology for both her undergraduate and master's degrees. She continued to doctoral studies at the same university where she completed her master's degree but was not able to complete the doctorate because politics and discriminatory treatment within the department became major obstacles to the continuation of her study. Even though she wants to live independently, she is living with her parents since it is too expensive to buy or rent a small apartment in Seoul, Korea. With her income, she is providing financial support for her parents while living with them.

Part I Encountering: "to come upon face to face"

Reconnecting with Hee-Yeon after 25 years

Hee-Yeon was my close childhood friend at the special education school for children with orthopedic impairments in Seoul, which we attended together for six years. After graduating from elementary school, we went on totally different life paths. We stayed in touch until we went to college and then lost contact. After about 25 years, we reconnected. While planning this book, I wondered how Hee-Yeon was doing. I had always believed she would be a successful and independent adult with her own career, and as I thought about recruiting participants, I hoped she would be a part of it. I looked for her on Facebook, and it was relatively easy to find her. I reached out via Facebook messenger, and like any other long-lost friends, we met at a coffee shop and shared stories about our lives since our college years. When I shared my idea for this project with her, Hee-Yeon was very excited to be a part of it. Her participation in this project is very special, and I feel honored to share her story.

Before we met up again, after so many years of not having talked with each other, I was a little worried that I would not be able to understand her speech. But I was very surprised that I was able to completely understand her speech. During the interviews, I shared my initial concern with Hee-Yeon and jokingly said, "I think sometimes I pretend to understand your speech." To this remark, she responded, "I know when people are pretending to understand my speech. I know you can understand my speech."

Hee-Yeon grew up in a lower-middle-class family. Her parents ran a small convenience store in the neighborhood where she attended middle and high school. They were busy working, and due to the age gap between Hee-Yeon and her brother, they were also busy taking care of him when she was attending school. Naturally, she was given more opportunities to be independent at an early age. For example, she had no choice but to learn to commute by herself from home to the elementary school via public transportation. Typically, in Korea, many children at the upper elementary school age are allowed to take public transportation on their own:

> Starting when I was in fifth grade, I took a taxi to school in the mornings. So it has been a long time since I began to commute by myself. I took the city bus for my commute back home. I think my mom picked me up at the bus station until I was in fifth grade. Do you remember, Yoon Joo? Your mom often gave me a ride to the bus station when she picked you up in the afternoon. Also, sometimes, teachers gave me rides to the bus station.

Because of her practice of commuting during elementary school, Hee-Yeon quickly learned how to be independent early on. During the first interview, as we were catching up and reminiscing about our childhood experiences, I realized there were many parts of her life that I had not really known about. I thought I knew a lot about Hee-Yeon's childhood, but as we shared our experiences, there were complex layers that I saw now as an adult. Her account of her commutes made me think about how her family dynamic and socioeconomic background created situations for her to be more proactive and independent despite challenges. The interview process helped rekindle our friendship and was very meaningful as we were able to reflect together on how our lived experiences of disability have evolved over time. The reflections and life stories Hee-Yeon shared during the three interviews were insightful, honest, raw, and thought-provoking, exceeding my initial expectations.

Experiencing physical barriers and negative stereotypes in educational settings

After graduating from elementary school, Hee-Yeon attended middle and high school in a mainstream setting. She was the only girl with disabilities among nondisabled students, and the transition from the special education school to the mainstream setting was very difficult for her in the beginning:

> The most challenging moment in my childhood was right after we graduated from the special education elementary school and transferred to middle school. It was 1987, the year we entered middle school. Back then, it was challenging for students with disabilities to enroll in mainstream public schools. I had to put all my energy into adjusting to the new environment. Also, the middle school I was assigned to happened to be the worst in the district, so not many students were interested in their studies.

The first obvious challenge for Hee-Yeon was the physical barrier. The middle school she attended was an old building with a lot of stairs and was located on the top of a high hill:

> I thought to myself, "At least I am able to walk." But for my first year of middle school, I was assigned to a classroom on the third floor. I still remember how difficult it was to climb all those steps with my backpack on. Keeping up with my studies was so challenging that I thought I was going to die.

Hee-Yeon not only faced physical barriers but was also not given equal access to all aspects of the curriculum. She studied very hard and studied in advance certain subjects, such as English, before the school year began. Her scores in language arts were in the top percentile, and her grades in many academic subjects were not bad. However, she faced barriers in certain subjects, and her "work hard" attitude could not resolve the challenges. For example, as a part of the high school entrance exam, students were required to take a physical fitness test. Out of 200 total points, 20 points were allocated to the physical fitness test:

> Since there were not enough students with disabilities in the past who took high school entrance tests, no scoring systems or accommodation procedures in physical fitness tests were in place for students with disabilities like me. Twenty points out of 200 was a significant portion, but

> unfortunately, I didn't get any accommodations for that. I thought it's a shame that there was nothing in place.

She further elaborated that music classes, which involved singing tests, were also difficult for her. Since she had significant articulation issues in her speech, she could not sing and participate with her classmates in their homeroom choir. In many middle and high schools in Korea, a major annual school event was a music festival in which choirs from different homerooms came together in a competition meant to promote a sense of unity and community among each homeroom. These anecdotes illustrate how Hee-Yeon was placed in mainstream settings full-time, but there were significant barriers at the systematic level that hindered her from fully integrating, and she could not do anything about them. These were moments of exclusion and marginalization.

Hee-Yeon has a mild physical disability and can walk and do most physical tasks independently. However, because her cerebral palsy affects her speech significantly, her disability is visible in many aspects, and she has faced many negative stereotypes because of her speech impairment:

> Especially in Korean society, people tend to be disrespectful and treat you [people with disabilities] like a child. But they treat me differently and use honorifics in their speech when they find out what school [university] I attended.

During her first semester at the mainstream middle school, Hee-Yeon felt negative attitudes toward her, even from the teachers, until she proved she was able to achieve academically:

> Fortunately, I studied hard for the exams and did impress my teachers with my grades during the first semester. Before my official scores on these exams came out, some teachers had looked down on me. They didn't discriminate against me or ignore me bluntly or explicitly, but I could sense implicit bias in their behaviors, voices, and subtle looks toward me.

Even though Hee-Yeon did not deal with this type of discriminatory experience every year, because of her speech impairment, she faced both explicit and subtle moments of exclusion in educational settings throughout her schooling experience. While she was attending graduate school for the doctorate degree, she felt "a wall between myself and others":

> There was some unfair treatment in my graduate school. For example, some professors skipped my parts during presentations. Also, I got eliminated from the list of students receiving scholarships. In the graduate school I attended, the professors favored students who could help

> expand their research agenda and work hard with an obedient attitude. But in their eyes, I wasn't capable, so I was eliminated from the inner circle of the professors' favorites. This was one of the bigger reasons I stopped pursuing my studies.

The anecdotes Hee-Yeon shared illustrate how she encountered the reality of her own disabled body as she faced obvious and subtle moments of marginalization and oppression.

Showing resiliency in the face of discriminatory systematic barriers: looking through critical eyes

During the first interview, when I asked Hee-Yeon to identify the moment when she recognized herself as a person with disabilities, she said:

> I think I was always aware of it [my disabilities]. My parents always said to me, "You must study hard since you have a disability." So after hearing their comments many times, I always knew I was a person with disabilities. I knew it throughout my school years.

Hee-Yeon's significant articulation issue as well as her visible physical disability makes her stand out in a crowd. Especially because of her articulation issue, she has faced more instances of discrimination, her voice has been often silenced, and her access to certain opportunities has been denied. She shared the following anecdote from her doctorate study in graduate school:

Hee-Yeon: Initially I wanted to study historical sociology, but one of the professors in that program was fickle and erratic. I thought to myself, how bad can he be. But soon after I started my first semester in that program, an upperclassman called me over and said, "I'm sorry to say this but the professor gives you permission to take his course but requests that you restrain yourself from speaking out and don't say anything during class time."

Yoon Joo: The college professor? Did a professor who teaches in the graduate school say comments like that?

Hee-Yeon: Yes. And he requested for me not to disrupt the flow of the lecture or cause discomfort during his class at any time.

Yoon Joo: Did you receive any treatment like this from any professors while you were attending college for your undergraduate degree?

Hee-Yeon: Yes. But there were so many students in the undergraduate classes that students were rarely given opportunities to speak up during the lecture. But in the graduate classes, there were usually more times for active participation and discussions.

Yoon Joo: Did you have any similar experiences in high school?

Hee-Yeon: In high school, many teachers just ignored me.

Yoon Joo: So they wouldn't call on you or ask you to read aloud passages from the text?

Hee-Yeon: Nope.

In the midst of these challenges, Hee-Yeon continued to fight and figure out ways to find her own place and voice to speak up. She had a firm belief that academic success and achievement were important vehicles for her to become fully integrated and successful in Korean society even though she was not able to complete her doctorate degree:

> When people find out I attended one of the most well-known universities in Seoul, I can see the flicker of change in their eyes. That's when I realized that if I wanted to live and make a living in Korea, I needed to be and do more than others. I enjoy studying and pursuing higher education degrees, but I also had other motives [for continuing to graduate school]. Others might consider it vain or even arrogant, but I was desperate to do and be more. Thinking back, if I hadn't attended graduate school, I don't think I could have had a successful adult life like I do now.

One of Hee-Yeon's ways of expressing her disability identity is through writing. Similar to the other women in this book, Hee-Yeon has been involved in disability advocacy work for women with disabilities, and she has shared her lived experiences of disability through her writing for the nonprofit advocacy organization's newsletter. However, discussion of her experience in the organization made me think about how the voices of disabled individuals can be silenced and marginalized by the agenda of an organization. This is Hee-Yeon's reflection on her experience working with this organization:

> I always questioned why the agenda of this organization was more centered around what nondisabled activists had to say rather than the voices of individuals with disabilities. There was a sense of discrimination within. Like a subtle nuance of discrimination. . . . Back then, this organization was run by both part-time and full-time staff members. Many of the part-time staff were very smart and well-spoken college students who were attending prestigious universities such as Ewha Womans University and Seoul National University. So, their voices became louder in our organization, and gradually, they became the dominant voice, setting the agenda and being in charge when determining the themes for activities within the organization. Their ideas weren't bad. But their ideas were more centered on a feminist approach, and this was appropriate for our organization. But feminist ideology was more dominant in setting the agenda for this organization, before considering the theoretical framework of disability studies. To be honest, there were many meetings and seminars in which I didn't understand what was discussed. Discussions would involve a lot of academic jargon that

> I wasn't familiar with. I wondered if people with disabilities would be able to understand and accept the writing in books and columns with this type of language.

Despite being nondisabled volunteers, the staff determined the dominant discourse in setting agendas in the organization.

Hee-Yeon was still able to find ways to raise her own voice through her writing. She talked about her own development as a writer:

Hee-Yeon: The language I used was far from common language. When I sometimes read my work from back then, it is very different from my writing style now. Back then, I used a lot of academic jargon and terminology. It was deemed as "better."

Yoon Joo: Yes, that's how it is many times.

Hee-Yeon: But you've read some of my current writings. My writing style is no longer difficult to read.

Yoon Joo: Yes, you're very good at writing jargon-free essays.

Hee-Yeon: After writing a lot of essays that were difficult to read, my thoughts about writing changed. Regardless of how other writings are, I want what I write to be easily read by all people – even those without prior knowledge of disabilities. I've engraved that on my brain.

Hee-Yeon was able to refine her writing style over the years to articulate her perspective on her lived experience of disability to reach out to a wider audience of readers. It was very interesting for me to observe Hee-Yeon's extraordinary ability to talk about her experience through a critical perspective.

Part II Embracing: "accept or support willingly and enthusiastically"

Developing close and unexpected friendships

Like many typical teenagers, in middle and high school, Hee-Yeon made several friends, and her close relationships with them have continued into her adult life. She said, "My middle and high school life was pretty good. My favorite part of my high school experience was meeting my best friends. We still hang out and are close friends. It's already been 30 years." Her middle school and high school were known as some of the worst in the district, and it was assumed that many of the students were not interested in academics and were more interested in partying. Hee-Yeon talked about how some of these students, who were known as "nalrari" (날라리) at her school, were more kindhearted and treated her more genuinely compared to others who were on top of the class academically. In Korea, nalrari refers to middle and high school students who were not interested in studying at all but spent most of their time in socializing with friends. These nalrari friends were a negative influence on Hee-Yeon's academic life, but she remembers interactions with them fondly:

> In my second year of middle school, I sort of went astray. I didn't study much. Instead of studying, I went to see live performances of musical bands or live radio talk shows. Back then, middle and high school students were expected to focus only on studying in every waking moment. My teachers and parents were worried because they thought I, a model student, was hanging out with the wrong crowd. Thinking back, it was not a big deal. From my perspective, these students were fun to hang out with and genuinely treated me as their friend.

When I asked Hee-Yeon, "In what ways did they care for you with sincerity?" she answered:

> I met her [one of the "nalrari" students] during my first year in middle school. As I was struggling to adjust to the mainstream classroom during the very beginning of my first year in middle school, she would sit next to me to eat lunch with me, carry my bag, and look after me during many moments throughout the school day. Even though I was young, I had developed an intuition for distinguishing peers who sincerely helped me versus others who were forced by teachers to help me. Anyway, she happened to hang out with the crowd that wasn't very studious, and I naturally started hanging out with them too. It was fun! But before I met this group of friends, I ate alone and didn't have anyone to hang out with. All the students would walk home together, but I didn't have that opportunity to socialize since I lived so close to the school. I wasn't bullied, but I was painfully lonely.

Hee-Yeon identified this friend as one of the few individuals who had significantly influenced her life outside of her family. They have stayed in touch for almost 30 years even though they live far from each other. She is also the person who sparked her enjoyment in theater performances. This story illustrates how genuine friendships helped Hee-Yeon socially integrate into mainstream schools. It also shows that students considered to be in the "wrong crowd" in the perspectives of parents and teachers cannot be assumed to be negative influences. Hee-Yeon was embraced for who she was by those least expected and developed genuine friendships with them that have lasted a lifetime.

Building a social network and experiencing a typical passage into adult life

As Hee-Yeon grew older, she met different people in many informal contexts outside of school settings and built meaningful social networks. She identified one former upper-level student from college as someone who had a significant impact on her life. This individual was a researcher at the Korean

Culture and Tourism Institute. Hee-Yeon said this about the strong influence she had on her life:

> It isn't about her being the only one who had a direct influence, but rather through her, I was able to meet a variety of people working in different fields. She helped me realize how narrow my perspective of looking at the world had been. She knew so many people and was the type of person to whom people were naturally drawn. So, whenever I would hang out with her, I naturally met so many cool people from art- or theater-related fields. Until then I didn't have the opportunity to meet people from other fields, but through her, I got connected with different professionals, and we became good friends.

This group consisted of professionals who worked as researchers at agencies related to coordinating performances or cultural events. Hee-Yeon recollected how she became really close to them during a short three-day trip as they hung out together and talked over drinks. As a young adult, she was embraced by others for who she was as they socialized through drinking. She also said, "They all treat me very well. One friend from this group currently lives in Busan and is very close to me. When I visit her occasionally, she still treats me like a princess."

Drinking is a major part of modern Korean socialization, especially among adults. A large majority of Korean people regard drinking as a necessary element of social life. As is the case for typical young adults in Korea, drinking parties were fun occasions for Hee-Yeon to socialize with other people. When asked for a photo that represents who she is, she submitted the following picture of a glass of beer (Figure 2.2).

With this picture, Hee-Yeon explained:

> First of all, I like alcohol more than people expect. When people drink with me at a bar or a restaurant, many of them are very pleasantly surprised that I eat and drink well, get along well with people, talk a lot, etc. I heard so many comments like this from people who drank with me for the first time. They were amazed by how I kept myself together even when I drank a lot and went back home alone without any accidents.
>
> It's not that I don't get drunk. In Korea, typically, several people come together to drink alcohol. On these occasions, I try very hard to keep myself together and be aware of my surroundings from the start to end. But as soon as I get home, I totally loosen up and collapse at home. [In Korea] not all drinking parties are for pleasure and socialization. Some drinking occasions involve work and business, so some people feel forced to join these occasions out of obligation even if they don't want to go. But in my case, through these informal meetings that involve drinking with people, I have a great opportunity for them to get to know about me.

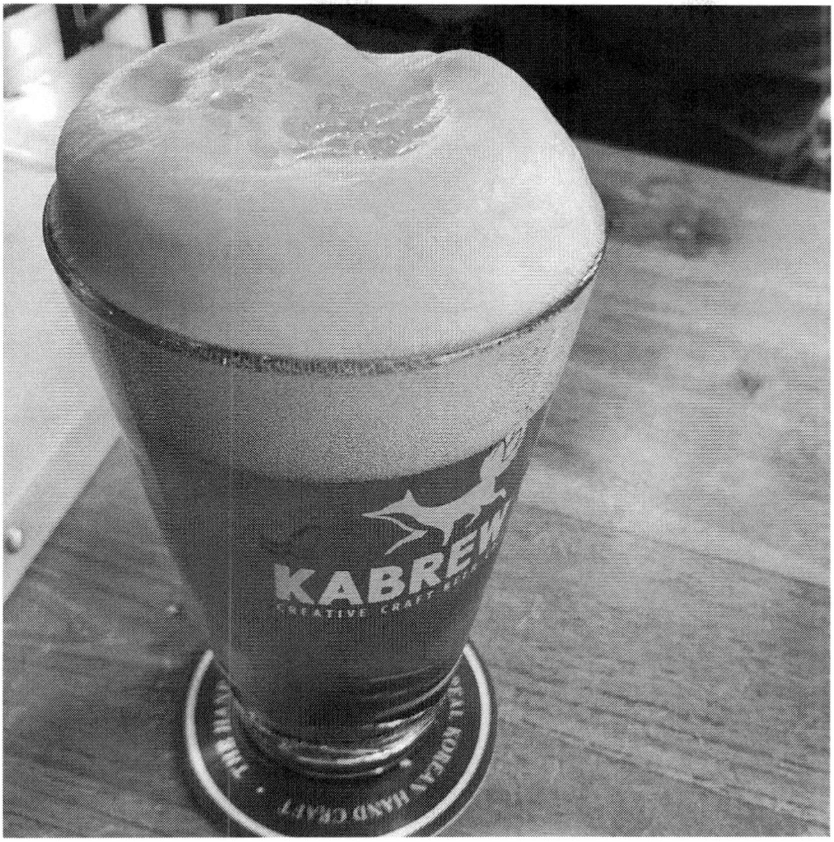

Figure 2.2 A glass of beer: symbolizing Hee-Yeon's journey of social connection

It is interesting to hear how Hee-Yeon was embraced as who she was and socially integrated in interpersonal contexts while she faced several kinds of discrimination in formal settings, such as graduate school. Her stories illustrate how she had very typical young adult experiences and social integration despite many marginalized experiences. In particular, informal gatherings for social drinking were an important vehicle for socialization in Hee-Yeon's life.

Part III Intersection of her story and my story

Looking back on our childhood in a segregated special education elementary school

I felt privileged to interview Hee-Yeon after so many years had passed. For the entire six years of elementary school, we both attended a special education school for children with physical and orthopedic disabilities. We conversed about many things and were able to share our memories. During the second interview, Hee-Yeon said, "It [the first interview] brought up a lot of memories from our elementary school days. I was amazed by how much I remembered. It has been *so* long, but I can still remember moments." Even though Hee-Yeon and I remembered different aspects, we both had fond memories of our days in the special education school:

Yoon Joo: Wasn't our school very nice? I don't remember how it was very well.
Hee-Yeon: It was the cleanest [compared to other special education schools].
Yoon Joo: Was it? I do remember thinking that the exterior was very pretty. The building was like The Little House on the Prairie.
Hee-Yeon: Yes. When I visited other places, I remember thinking how it looked strange to me when I saw some students' faces were a little bit messy and smelly. You know, in many cases, it's hard for some disabled children to maintain hygiene. But when I first visited our school, it was kept very clean, and there were no strange body odors. When I first started at the school as a first grader, I found it interesting that almost everyone at the school was much older or younger [than their grade level]. You were the only one the same age as I was. I think we were the only ones who were at the appropriate age corresponding to our grade.

It was interesting to me how Hee-Yeon's memories included smells of certain places. The special education school that we attended was hospital-affiliated and a lab school setting. Children in the school had annual check-ups with orthopedists in the hospital, and many students from several top universities did their internship, student teaching, and volunteer work in this school. Our conversation about this special education elementary school continued:

Hee-Yeon: Now that I think about it . . . those were the good old days.
Yoon Joo: We got to meet many volunteers who came to our school and taught us piano, violin, and calligraphy, right? I wanted to take violin lessons so badly but couldn't [because my right hand was too spastic to hold the violin steady].
Hee-Yeon: Thinking back, I feel like most children who attended our school came from upper-middle class. I guess there was a unique vibe, and the influence is still with me. There was a particular ambience that still influences me.
Yoon Joo: What kind of influence?
Hee-Yeon: My mom often says I was exposed to only nice things as a young child, and that's why I tend to spend money on buying good things. [laughs]
Yoon Joo: Ah, I see.

Hee-Yeon: This is 100% my opinion, but I feel like the school community was a little bit closed off. It was different from the rest of the world.

Yoon Joo: I guess it was kind of in its own bubble.

Hee-Yeon: I remember the community at the special education elementary school felt like a bubble and had a unique vibe and its own ambience, unlike other special education schools that I visited. While attending there, I only saw the good side of people. And I acted according to those standards. I didn't think about or suspect any bad intentions from others. I think some of that still lives within me. I think my relationships from there influenced how I relate to others in different social contexts and helped me to enjoy being around people.

Reflecting back on this conversation, I realized how this school setting was privileged, and many children from affluent families attended this school. It was almost a sheltered environment for children with disabilities. My mom shared with me how she decided to send me to this school because she observed how the teachers were nice and could trust them. Our school community had been a very important place for both Hee-Yeon and me, laying the foundations for our lives later on. The social network of children with physical disabilities was a foundational experience for us. Since all our elementary school friends had physical disabilities, we felt accepted as we were. Someone on the outside might object to this kind of environment as inappropriately segregated, but this experience helped us become more capable when we were finally mainstreamed. For me, in the beginning, mainstreaming was challenging, but whenever I faced difficulties, I remembered how well-regarded I had been in the academic and social network of the special education school. This helped me discern when my typically developing peers began to see me beyond my disability. Perhaps, paradoxically, the segregated environment was a foundation for social inclusion for me.

A unique issue emerged from Hee-Yeon's story: the intersection of SES and disability

My family's socioeconomic background is upper-middle class. My parents provided me with financial support to go through college and graduate schools without taking out student loans. For most of my life, I did not experience financial crisis. While I was reflecting on our elementary school experience with Hee-Yeon, I felt uncomfortable to a certain extent because I realized I had been in a position of privilege. I was surprised at how Hee-Yeon noticed differences between her experience and the experiences of many others who came from wealthy families. I had not really thought about whether someone had come from a rich family or not. Reflecting back, I realized how I was one of the privileged children, so I took many things granted. It was interesting that Hee-Yeon referred to the SES of classmates when she shared certain anecdotes:

Yoon Joo: Your story reminds me of a sad story about one of upper-level student.

Hee-Yeon: I remember him being very smart and diligent in his studies. I heard that he wanted to work in a computer related field, but there were no jobs for him. Back then, there weren't any social supports, policies, or laws [related to equal employment opportunities] in place. He was probably going through a lot. Something I've wondered about is. . . . I recall his family being financially well-off.

Yoon Joo: Yes, that's how I recall it too.

Hee-Yeon: I wonder why his family didn't think of sending him to study abroad.

Yoon Joo: Yes, I've wondered the same.

Hee-Yeon: He had a pretty severe physical disability but he was so smart. I feel like if his family had supported him a little . . . back then, it was better [to study abroad]. Back then, it was common for people with disabilities to study abroad if their families were financially doing well.

This story made me think back on the social climate of Korea in the 1990s for people with disabilities. If there had been less stigma toward people with disabilities, there would have been opportunities for people who had so much potential to achieve so much more in life. There were so many people who had great capacity but were left behind, without any support or resources. Hee-Yeon mentioned several times that she would like to have studied abroad because "people tended to look down upon me" because of her visible disabilities in speech and walking. She explained her desire to study abroad and live in another country outside of Korea:

> I can't say it was a motivation. It's kind of funny. Well, 50% of the reason [I wanted to study abroad] was because I enjoyed pursuing my studies. The other 50% was [general perspectives toward people with disabilities] in Korea. If an individual has a disability, especially communication/speech challenges, and on top of that, the individual is a female, she has nowhere to go after graduating from college. I can't speak for how it might have changed now, but back then, it was impossible [for a woman with disabilities] to find a job.

However, Hee-Yeon could not go abroad:

> I had a few complications in life so I stopped pursuing my PhD after a year, and then I had a plan to study abroad. The plan was to study in

> Germany because it was common for students whose major was sociology to go study in Germany. But while I was preparing for study abroad, my family had a major financial crisis, so I had to work.

Hee-Yeon's story reminded me of how disability is a multivariant construct that is experienced intersectionally. During the interviews, she articulated clearly how her lived experiences have been impacted by not only the visible nature of her disability but also her gender and her family's socioeconomic background. Her family lived in a part of Seoul where the public schools were not appropriated equipped to integrate students with disabilities. This affected Hee-Yeon's middle and high school experiences. Also her family did not have financial means to support her for the advanced degree. This impacted the range of possible job opportunities for Hee-Yeon. Hee-Yeon and I might have similar capacities to succeed, but our lived experiences evolved differently because of our family's socioeconomic background. SES encompasses resources for further educational opportunities and financial security as well as privileges and quality of life attributes. Hee-Yeon clearly has the capacity and motivation to advance her educational career to elevate her social status through studying abroad but was unable to do so because of lack of financial support. Also, she is clearly able to live alone out of her parents' house as a typical adult; however, it is financially challenging for her to afford a place of her own because housing price in Seoul Korea is very high. Yet she was able to successfully accomplish in her life as a full-time editor in a field that does not easily open the doors to individuals with disabilities. It is important to remember that disability is not a single factor but multiple factors such as SES complicate the quality of life in the lived experiences of individuals with disabilities across life span.

3 Jinju

Living in the body of a disabled person with the perspective of a nondisabled person

> 장애인 인걸 잊어버릴 때는 없는 것 같아요. 저는 제가 장애인 인 것은 너무 당연한 사실이라고 생각을 해서 받아드려서, 내가 할 수 있는 것과 할 수 없는 것의 경계는 되게 명확했던 것 같아요. 내가 못한다고 해서 그게 우울하거나 절망적이지는 않았던 것 같아요. 내가 가고 싶은 곳을, 예를 들어서 내가 액티비티 같은 것을 못해서 비장애인처럼 그렇게 역동적인 활동들을 못해서 내가 장애가 없었으면 저런걸 할 수 있었을텐데, 막 저런 것 하고 싶다- 하고 싶은 마음이 간절했다면 제 장애를 비관할 수도 있었겠죠. 그런데 그렇게 하고 싶은 마음이 ㅎㅎㅎ 없었고, 그냥 내가 살아가고 있는 이 길이 굉장히 즐거웠고 행복했었기 때문에 ㅎㅎㅎ 제 장애가 크게 걸림돌이 됐었던 것 같지도 않고, 크게 내 인생에 영향을 미치는 것 같지도 않고 그래서 장애가 크게 다가오지도 않고, 그러니까 그래서 그런지 장애인인건 너무 당연한데, 그렇다고 해서 내가 장애인 인 것을 잊어먹고, 아 나 장애인. 가끔 친구들이랑 놀다보면 친구들 입에서 "아 우리 장애인이지"라고 하기는 해요. 친구들이랑 막 수다 떨고 놀다보면 "아 그래 우리 장애인이야" 뭐 이러기는 농담처럼 하기는 하는데 . . . .
>
> [I don't think I ever forget that I am a person with a disability. I've accepted my disability to the point where I automatically think that it is a part of me. I clearly recognize the things I can do and cannot do because of my physical disabilities. I've never been sad or depressed because of the fact that I cannot do certain things. If I wished I were born with a normal body and wanted to do certain things, go to different places, as well as do certain activities, perhaps I would feel sad and devastated. But I've never had that kind of pessimistic mindset. I just feel content and happy with who I am. I do enjoy my life as it is, and my disability doesn't feel like a very big obstacle in my life. I don't think my disability was a big tragedy in my life. I just accept my disabled body as it is, and it is who I am even though I cannot forget the fact that I am a person with physical disabilities. Sometimes when I hang out with my friends with disabilities, we just make jokes like "Yay, right, we are people with a disability" . . . .]
>
> – Jinju

Jinju is a 40-year-old woman with Laing distal myopathy, the severest of the physical challenges experienced by the four women in this book. Laing distal

DOI: 10.4324/9781003609179-3

myopathy is a very rare degenerative muscle disorder. Characteristics of this disability include weakness in the feet and ankles, followed by weakness in the hands and wrists. Jinju's spinal cord is not straight, so her body posture is atypical, her muscles have slowly stiffened, and her joints, such as in the ankles or knees, are distorted. She uses a special wheelchair that was made just for her to support her body position, and she needs physical assistance in many areas for her to carry out daily functions. However, her disability does not affect her speech and cognitive abilities.

Jinju was born and raised in South Korea. She was the only child in a two-parent household. She grew up in a upper-middle-class family. During the interview, she shared how her family environment was nurturing and privileged, thanks to her father's financial support and her mother's dedication to advocate for Jinju's education. She talked about the tremendous dedication and support her parents had provided her with:

> My parents never hid me away at home. Rather, they would become my hands and legs and take me wherever they could so that I was able to be exposed to a variety of experiences. Every summer, my father took us on vacation to different places in Korea. Thinking back, even though I am their only child, there must've been so much to prepare and care for, given my disability. Regardless, every year, they packed a ton of stuff for a vacation that lasted only a few days and few nights. They told me, "Jinju, since we need to go places with appropriate accommodations for you, we can't go camping but we can go to hotels and motels all over the country." So just like that, we traveled to all different places, such as every historical site in the textbooks I studied at school, the East Sea coast one year and the South Sea coast the next. We really went to all the places in Korea. Therefore, despite my disability, I feel like I've been everywhere and have experienced everything, even more than my friends without disabilities. In that aspect, I had more opportunities to experience a variety of places that widened my perspective. My parents gifted me these experiences and showered me with love that perhaps a typical child might not be able to experience. How my parents treated me truly showed me how much they love me and through that I felt happiness.

Jinju only attended mainstream schools from the elementary school to the university. She is a disability advocate and has worked in a nonprofit Christian-affiliated social welfare research institute. For her undergraduate degree, she studied social welfare and completed her doctorate degree in this area. At the time I interviewed her for this project, she had completed all the coursework in her doctoral program and was working on her dissertation. While she was writing her dissertation, she was working two days a week at the research institute. Her job was to participate in assigned research projects. Within the organization, she was also considered a good point person to promote disability awareness, so she served as a disability advocate, giving speeches to people and organizations to raise awareness of disability-related issues and working on YouTube content regarding disability awareness.

In her twenties, she lived alone in a small apartment in a city an hour away from Seoul and was physically more active. In her special wheelchair, she traveled abroad alone without her parents several times. She visited New Zealand to attend an eight-week language program and participated in a short missionary program to Thailand, China, and Japan with the professors at her university. She also traveled to the United States with a few fellow students for a sister language program at the University of Mississippi for four weeks. But, at one point in her thirties, she experienced severe anemia and was hospitalized for several weeks. After dealing with the major health crisis, she moved back to living with her mom.

Because of her significant physical challenges, she needs services from a disability support worker in terms of transportation as well as daily living tasks. In Korea, disability support workers provide care services for people with significant disabilities. Jinju shared how difficult it is to get matched with the right disability support worker because there are not enough people well trained for this job:

> For people who are very ill and bedridden, a caregiver needs to change the body position once in a while to prevent bed sores, assist with feeding, and use machines or diapers for bathroom needs so it might be easier to commit long term. On the other hands, active people with severe disabilities like me, the caregivers are required to use a great amount of strength throughout the day such as lifting me up to seat me in the toilet. In the past, my muscles weren't as weak, so I could go to the bathroom on my own, and the caregiver would help me with simple house chores. At that time, I was able to keep the same caregiver for at least a year or two. However, as my body weakened, I have more physical needs such as carrying me out of the shower and wiping the wet floor in the bathroom before taking the shower, as well as helping me more in and out of my wheelchair. I am not trying to be picky in selecting a caregiver. But some caregivers are hesitant when I share all my specific needs during the interview. So it has been hard finding a caregiver.

At the time of the interview, she was searching for a new disability support worker but was having hard time finding one. Because she was not able to find the right support worker, her mom was helping her with many tasks. Despite some challenges, she continues to try her best, living her daily life as a student and working professional.

Part I Encountering: "to come upon face to face"

Meeting Jinju for the first time

I invited Jinju to participate in this project after watching YouTube clips of her speaking at several events during disability awareness week in Korea. I was intrigued by how she clearly articulated her experience of living with the perspective of a nondisabled individual was interesting, so I decided to reach out to her for the interviews. Even though I was a complete stranger to her, she was very open to participating in my project. After a quick phone call and a few introductory email exchanges, I conducted three interviews with her via Zoom. Because I was not familiar with her disability, I started the first interview by asking about her early experiences and educational history to get to know more about the extent to which her physical disabilities affected different aspects of her life.

During the first interview, Jinju shared that she spent many months during her infancy and toddler years in the hospital undergoing therapies and exercises. During her toddler years, her parents hoped she would walk alongside other children and were desperate to help her body become physically normal, so they agreed to the doctor's recommendation to try a new technique, surgeries that would cut her Achilles and pierce the knee so they could bend in the correct direction. She went through several surgeries, and every time, her muscles became further stiffened as a result of having a cast on for extended periods. The doctors would do physical rehabilitation therapy to address the stiff muscles, but her bones were too fragile and often broke. This led to another vicious round of putting on the cast and physical therapy. From when she was about 100 days old until she turned 4, she was hospitalized many times. She commented on this early memory:

> Whenever I see something white, it reminds me of the hospital – the white gown, the white hat the nurses wore, and the entire hospital was a world of white. That is one of my earliest memories, the white world and being terrified of it.

Before Jinju entered preschool, her parents realized her disability was not a disease that could be "cured," and before she entered elementary school, her parents had to make an important decision:

> My parents' minds flooded with many thoughts: "Do we send her to a special education school or public mainstream school?" "Do we have the option of sending her to a public school?" "Would the school accept her enrollment?" Back then, it was uncommon for a child with disabilities to be enrolled in a mainstream classroom at a public school.

Her parents were worried because it was very common for public schools to blatantly reject enrollment of children with disabilities. However, when they noticed she did not have any cognitive delays and knew she was capable of following a general education curriculum in a public school, they decided to enroll her in a mainstream school:

> Sending me to a special school might be the easier route in the short run, but thinking about it in the long term, they [Jinju's parents] thought the seclusion from other students without disabilities could hinder my life as an adult after graduation from school. In order to prepare me to be part of society, my parents made the ultimate decision that they would advocate for me to attend a mainstream preschool, elementary school, middle school, and high school.

In many aspects of Jinju's life, her parents made sure she was given all the help she needed to succeed. It was clear her parents had positively influenced her life.

Because I was not familiar with Jinju's physical disabilities at all, in the beginning, I asked a lot of questions related to her daily routine as well as her physical conditions. It was hard for me to picture her physical movements in spaces since all the interviews occurred in Zoom. I noticed myself feeling conscious and cautious about whether or not I was asking inappropriate questions related to her physical conditions. Even though I also have a physical disability, I have a certain level of anxiety and discomfort because I was not familiar with her disability. I am grateful that Jinju openly shared her conditions answering all my questions. A month after our three Zoom interviews, we were able to meet in person. She came all the way to a restaurant near my parents' house to see me. Arranging an in-person meeting with an individual in a wheelchair was an interesting process for me. Since Jinju suggested that she come to my neighborhood, I had to think hard to come up with wheelchair accessible places, and it took me a while to decide on a meeting place. When I met her in person, I got a more concrete sense of how physical challenges might impact Jinju's life. Even though I was also a person with physical disabilities, to a certain degree, I was uncomfortable seeing the physical challenges associated with her disabled body. Her physical presence was quite noticeable in the public space (a restaurant) where we shared our meal and had a typical fellowship. My meeting with Jinju was an eye-opening experience for me since the extents of our disabilities were very different.

Encountering her disabled body: being left behind

From elementary school to high school, Jinju was the only girl with disabilities among all of the other nondisabled students in the mainstream setting. While Jinju was in school, she was generally independent regarding academic-related tasks, for example, taking her own notes. But she needed help with moving around in the school building. She asked friends for piggyback rides during break times to grab snacks or to hang out with friends. Except for help with mobility, she did not receive any other assistance. Overall, Jinju thought she was well-integrated socially with her peers:

> I had awesome friends and teachers throughout my schooling experiences. When the homeroom teachers treated me without discrimination, the students naturally treated me the same way. Classmates approached me first, and we quickly became friends. Sometimes, they had to play Rock, Paper, Scissors because too many friends wanted to help me. Most students were kind and caring, but there were always a few exceptions. For example, a kid once said to me, "Hey, retard," and another, "You can't even walk. Try to catch me." They were mostly immature boy classmates, and there were at least two or three of them every year. But my mom always helped me process the situations I had experienced so I was never permanently traumatized by these events.

Even in an environment where she was socially well-integrated, Jinju faced situations in which she was not completely a part of the typical school experience. During the first two years of elementary school, her homeroom teacher made an effort to include her during the PE period. The teacher brought her to the gym and had her hold on to the bench so she could stand and observe the other students. Although the teacher's actions may have been considerate and good-intentioned, they did not create a meaningful experience for Jinju. She was still on the margins, feeling lost:

> I never knew what was going on. For example, when they were playing kickball, the teacher explained the rules, format of the game, etc. But since they were too far away, I couldn't hear any of the rules. From my viewpoint, they were just mindlessly kicking the ball, so I lost interest.

Jinju shared how she stopped going to the gym to observe other students and stayed in the classroom during PE. She did not mind staying in the classroom while the others were at gym or on the playground:

> Classmates gave me their valuables such as Walkmans, CD players, and MP3 players to keep safe. I could see that some of them felt guilty as they suggested I listen to the songs they had on their devices. So during PE, I stayed back in the classroom, listening to music, reading books, and such.

These stories illustrate how kindness and good intentions from nondisabled peers and teachers were not the magic solution for Jinju to be fully integrated into every aspect of a typical everyday school experience. On the surface, she was placed in an inclusion environment with nondisabled peers for the whole school day. At the same time, it is clear she was not completely a part of all the opportunities. She recalled these events fondly without any resentment or negative feelings and accepted them as they were.

Building mutual and meaningful relationships

Jinju was dependent upon other peers to move between different parts of the school. While attending an all-girls middle school, in some ways she felt more comfortable asking peers for piggyback rides when she had to transition to another classroom for art or music. Because Jinju had to rely on her peers in this aspect, this affected the nature of her relationships with them. Jinju talked about how her relationship with a close friend became complicated and how she had to deal with subtle nuances in their relationship dynamics:

> At first, most of my classmates had a genuine intention to help me, but as teachers began to compliment them, those classmates became more aware of this. The teachers would say, "Wow, so-and-so is helping Jinju. Great job," and at first, the friends responded, "Oh, thank you." However, as more of my friends helped me, people started referring to me as the one who always needs help. One friend who helped me the most often slowly became my designated helper. She was the role model who always helped the friend with the disability, and soon, I became her responsibility. Even on days she wasn't feeling well, like when she was on her period, she still felt obligated to help me. More and more, she became agitated easily, and there was a subtle tension between us. It would have been better if it had been just for one year, but the following year, that friend's mom volunteered for my friend to be placed in the same class as me. The teachers happily agreed, thinking it would be best to have a familiar friend with me. In the first year, my friend had only the best intentions, but the second year was very different. I could tell she felt obligated and was no longer sincere. I started to resent her for that. From her perspective, I was the ungrateful one. When I told this to my mom, she agreed that I sometimes even took her for granted. This is one of my unhappy memories. A part of me thinks of it as a lesson learned. After this experience, I kindly asked my friends to take turns helping me. Although I was always grateful for any help, I explained that I did not want anyone to feel obligated or designated to help me. I even joked that I would like to be given piggyback rides by different people, not just one. Through a not-so-happy memory, I learned how to communicate with friends and develop more social skills to navigate relationship dynamics that can be complicated sometimes.

Jinju went through a steep learning curve to develop healthy boundaries with her nondisabled peers. She needed to negotiate with her social network for physical assistance to be transported across different rooms. She clearly needed a significant measure of help from friends to survive in a mainstream setting as an individual with disabilities. At the same time, she had to go through an intricate process to maintain a mutual friendship in which she was not someone who needed help all the time. She had to go through an extra layer of personal reflection, requiring self-efficacy skills to assert herself as an equal partner.

Friendship plays a significant part in one's childhood and youth. As one comes to adulthood, romantic relationships, in addition to friendships, bring important meaning to one's life. When I asked Jinju about a time when she was more aware of her disability, she answered:

> There was a moment of recognition I had toward my disability. When I was in my twenties, I was once madly in love. It was the first and last time I was truly in love. In the past, I'd had crushes and short flings, more like puppy love. But at that time, it was different. We did everything other normal couples would do, including showing physical affection. I was in my twenties and I really liked the guy. When he was sick, I loved him so much that I wanted to hurt instead of him. But because of my disability, I found myself unable to take care of him physically. I couldn't take him to the hospital or pick up his medicine at the pharmacy. I yearned to do what lovers do for each other, like what I saw in TV dramas, like cooking a surprise meal for their sick boyfriend and such. However, in reality, I couldn't do any of it as someone with disabilities. One day, we were on a date, and he was running a dangerously high fever. We decided to call a cab to go to the hospital, but it was going to take too long to catch a wheelchair friendly cab. Since it was an emergency situation, I stopped a regular cab on the street, and he had to go ahead to the hospital by himself. By the time I had arrived at the hospital, it was several hours later, and he had already received treatment and was sent home. At that moment, I really realized the impact of my disabled body. If I hadn't had my disability, I could have done so much more for him. It was a recognition that wasn't pleasant at all.

When Jinju shared this anecdote, I completely understood where she was coming from. Even though I felt comfortable openly discussing my own disability experiences in other contexts, I was reluctant to address the topic of intimate dating relationships. As a woman with physical disabilities, I was hesitant and uncomfortable talking about dating because I assumed dating was not appropriate for me. I developed the blind expectation that my physical disability was a major imperfection that men could not accept and that they would not perceive me as an attractive romantic partner. Fearing rejection in a dating relationship, I chose and tried my best to adopt a nonsexual lifestyle. I avoided any kind of dating situations and shied away from actively seeking a romantic relationship even though my desires were strong and real.

For women with physical disabilities, more than any other social context, romantic relationships make them hyperaware of their disabled body and lead to the feeling of being "not good enough" as a partner.

Part II Embracing: "accept or support willingly and enthusiastically"

Rediscovering disability identity through friendships with other disabled peers

Jinju attended a private Christian university in a city two hours from Seoul, the capital of South Korea, for her undergraduate degree. This university is known for providing students with disabilities with access to a college education. The criteria for admission are more flexible, and a wide range of services are available for students with disabilities. Compared to other universities in Korea, there are a relatively larger number of disabled students attending this university. Jinju mentioned her college experience was meaningful and valuable in reexamining how she viewed herself as an individual with disabilities as well as those with other disabilities that were different from hers. Jinju shared a specific exchange she had with her best friend Theresa (Chapter 4) during college that was an eye-opening experience for her own level of disability awareness:

> One day, I was commenting to a friend [Theresa] half-jokingly, "You're stupid. How can you not know that?" She felt my joke was very insulting and was very hurt by the fact that I called her "stupid." She could have broken off our friendship and simply stopped talking to me. However, thankfully, when I persistently asked her why she was upset about my joking comment, she explained she often felt inferior to me. When I asked, "Why do you feel inferior?" she replied, "You attended a mainstream school. I had to go to a special education school." Shocked and puzzled, I said, "So what?" She explained the scope and sequence of curriculum at special education schools were limited and less challenging compared to regular schools, and many of the "extra" classes, such as learning Chinese characters, were excluded, leaving the students who want to learn to be self-taught. In her special education school, the classes focused on therapeutic aspects such as physical therapy rather than academics, and there was minimal support for preparing for the college entrance exam. Therefore, differences were inevitable, and she felt I had poked fun at what she had been deprived of. Up to this point, I had been a little bit immature and didn't see the whole picture. That's one of the moments when I realized I had lived with the perspective of a nondisabled person to that point.

Even though both Jinju and her friend have physical disabilities, their perspectives and responses in certain situations were different because of their educational experiences prior to college. Jinju is fully appreciative of her experience in mainstream settings, she also acknowledges uniquely empowering opportunities that only occur in special education schools:

> As I began to reflect on my school years, I realized that I had also missed out in other ways of being an active participant while attending a mainstream school. For example, I didn't have access to any of therapeutic programs like physical therapy to fix my posture or provide me with appropriate exercises. I was the classroom keeper during PE. I had assumed I was incapable of participating in PE class. But friends who attended a special education school told me there were sports people with disabilities could play, such as Boccia. When I asked, "What is Boccia?," they replied, "It's a sport people with disabilities can do. You roll a ball on something that looks like a slide." I thought, "Hey, I can do that," and when I did, I had so much fun. I also began to question myself, "Why hadn't I known this before?"

Through a social network of other individuals with various disabilities during her college years, Jinju was challenged to examine her own assumptions about other people with disabilities and make sense of her disabled body in different ways as she interacted with her disabled peers:

> Although I knew those students had gone through the application process just like I had, there were times throughout conversations where I felt like I knew more than them [due to attending a mainstream school].
>
> People with disabilities are portrayed though a biased perspective in the Korean media. When thinking about people with hearing or visual impairments, there is a prejudice because of the biases from the media. I was no exception until I actually met other students at the university. I started to learn sign language and realized truly how to socialize with people with visual impairments. One day, Theresa shared that she had applied for a helping aide position at the disability center at our university. I asked, "How in the world are you going to help others with disabilities when you have one yourself?" She answered, "I can help type up lectures and help with transitioning from one class to another." Puzzled, I asked, "You're in a wheelchair, how will you help them with transitioning between classrooms?" She replied, "I can have a blind person hold onto my wheelchair handles as I lead the way." So that's when I first realized people with disabilities can help other disabled individuals. I had always received help from nondisabled peers, and that is all I knew and never thought to challenge my own abilities. These are things I learned not through coursework but from personal experiences I had the opportunity to absorb during my 4 years in college.

Jinju's stories reveal how her perspective toward other disabled individuals is closely connected to how she views her own disabilities. Her narratives also clearly illustrate how people's experiences of disability may be different depending on their educational background. Jinju was very articulate when she reflected on how her perspective was different from that of her disabled peers who attended the special education school. Her story illustrates the importance of being in a community with other individuals with disabilities.

Embracing a moment of challenge and turning it into a major milestone

Her four-year college experience of living in a dorm apart from her parents was the major milestone in Jinju's journey of embracing her disability, specifically, in terms of establishing independence as a grown adult. Because of the significant impact of her physical limitations on daily living, it is important to consider what having an independent life meant to her. When she was first accepted to university, Jinju and her parents contemplated finding a place where her mother could live with her. But her parents thought it was important for her to utilize the resources that the university provided to support people with disabilities so she would not become dependent on her mother:

> They [Jinju's parents] believed it was important for me to experience living independently, hanging out with friends, and problem solving through daily challenges. When my parents and I made the decision for me to live in the dorms, the school, at first, said it would be difficult to provide that option. Then my parents made a deal with the school, offering to provide a scholarship to a student who would be assigned as my roommate and help me with my daily living in the dorm. Furthermore, they requested to be anonymous donors so that the student with financial needs could accept the role with the pure intention to help and a desire to study. So the school found a student that needed the scholarship and was willing to help.

Jinju described how this arrangement turned out differently than expected:

> This arrangement backfired because the student had a bigger financial need and needed to work other part-time jobs to earn money for her daily living expenses as well as send home money to support her family. In the beginning, she was not fully informed of the details concerning the conditions under which the scholarship was given – that she would have to help me around the dorm. For example, I expected her to help me in the shower after her classes, but she went straight to her part-time job. I remember not being able to shower for an entire week once. This happened during my first semester of my first year in college.

Jinju further explained her roommate was not neglecting her duty or intentionally mistreating her, and that this event brought a pleasantly surprising outcome:

> On weekends, she left to go home and help out her family, but I had to stay behind to study for exams. After not being able to shower for a week, I couldn't stand it. So I grabbed the back scratcher I brought around to help me reach things and used it to undress myself. It was inconvenient and uncomfortable, but after 2 hours I had showered all by myself. After that experience, I became more independent while I was living in the dorm. I no longer automatically asked for help and received help for only the things I absolutely could not do on my own. I used my electric wheelchair to go to class on my own and wrote my own notes per usual. Besides the times I woke up late and required a bit of support to get to class on time, I was independent. Because that student was too busy to help me, I learned to do things on my own. My parents saw this in a positive light and told me that it was meant to be and to be grateful it happened this way. They continued to provide her with a scholarship for her studies. One day, the student asked me, "What is your father's name?" And I told her. Then she realized that her scholarship was being provided by my family, not the university. She said she felt bad to accept such a big amount of money when she couldn't do much for me. So I told her, "You were not intentionally refusing to help me. You didn't have time for your own good reasons and responsibilities. Through that, I grew independent, and both my parents and I are grateful for that." We are friends and still keep in touch.

As she went through this experience, Jinju became more independent and was even able to travel abroad alone to attend a short-term language program:

> The first time I traveled without my parents, it was just me and my wheelchair on the plane to New Zealand for an 8-week language program. Then I went on a short missionary program to Thailand, China, and Japan with the professors from my school. I also traveled to America with a few fellow students for a sister language program at the University of Mississippi for 4 weeks.

After graduating from college, she lived independently in a small apartment since her parents had moved to the countryside. Recalling those times, she said, "I felt confident in living alone and looking back, they were the most delightful days of my life":

> This section illustrates how she embraced her disability identity through the recognition of challenges as well as through moments of discovery.

> My disability is "my plus alpha" [added benefit], adding many positive things to my life. I always include this motto when I talk about myself on college and graduate school applications and resumes. It has become the biggest part of my identity that developed into who I am today. My mother planted this positive outlook in me, and then I developed it into my own philosophy and beliefs. It started with how I perceive my own disability. And then this is connected to how people with disabilities view one another and how others may perceive my disability. All of these things I have shared during my lectures for disability awareness.

Embracing the life of a disabled body in a very special wheelchair and opening the door to many possibilities

During the interviews, I asked Jinju to talk about an important person in her life outside of her family who had supported her and had a positive influence on her. She identified the man who developed her custom wheelchair. As Jinju's disability affects her body posture and sitting positions, she needs a special wheelchair to support her body. However, she cannot use the typical wheelchairs that many individuals with disabilities use, and needs a custom-made wheelchair (Figures 3.1 and 3.2).

She talked about how her wheelchair was an important representation of who she is:

> My wheelchair is not an ordinary wheelchair, and it has become my mascot. My wheelchair was customized for my body and made to address my needs as a student. The creator of my wheelchair took into consideration what I needed as a college student, such as a desk with a lid that has a compartment so I can put in books I need to carry to class.
>
> Usually on the street, if people see someone in a regular wheelchair, they would probably remember the encounter. Therefore, I really leave a strong impression since my wheelchair does not look like a typical wheelchair, and many people remember me easily. Sometimes I wonder if people would be as interested in me if I used a typical wheelchair. I ask myself, "Would it look very different from what I have now?" "Would it change the quality of my life?" My current wheelchair can also work as a convenient introduction. For example, when I make a phone call to a new place for work and introduce myself with "Hello, this is Jinju, a researcher from the Social Welfare Center," the person on the other side of the phone call usually does not remember me at first. But when I remind the person, "I'm the one that has the really unique wheelchair," the person would respond, "Ah . . . yes, I remember you now." So my wheelchair has truly become a part of my identity as well as my mascot. It represents me and describes me. I also talk about my wheelchair during the lectures on disability awareness, and this topic is a unique way to introduce myself easily to the audience.

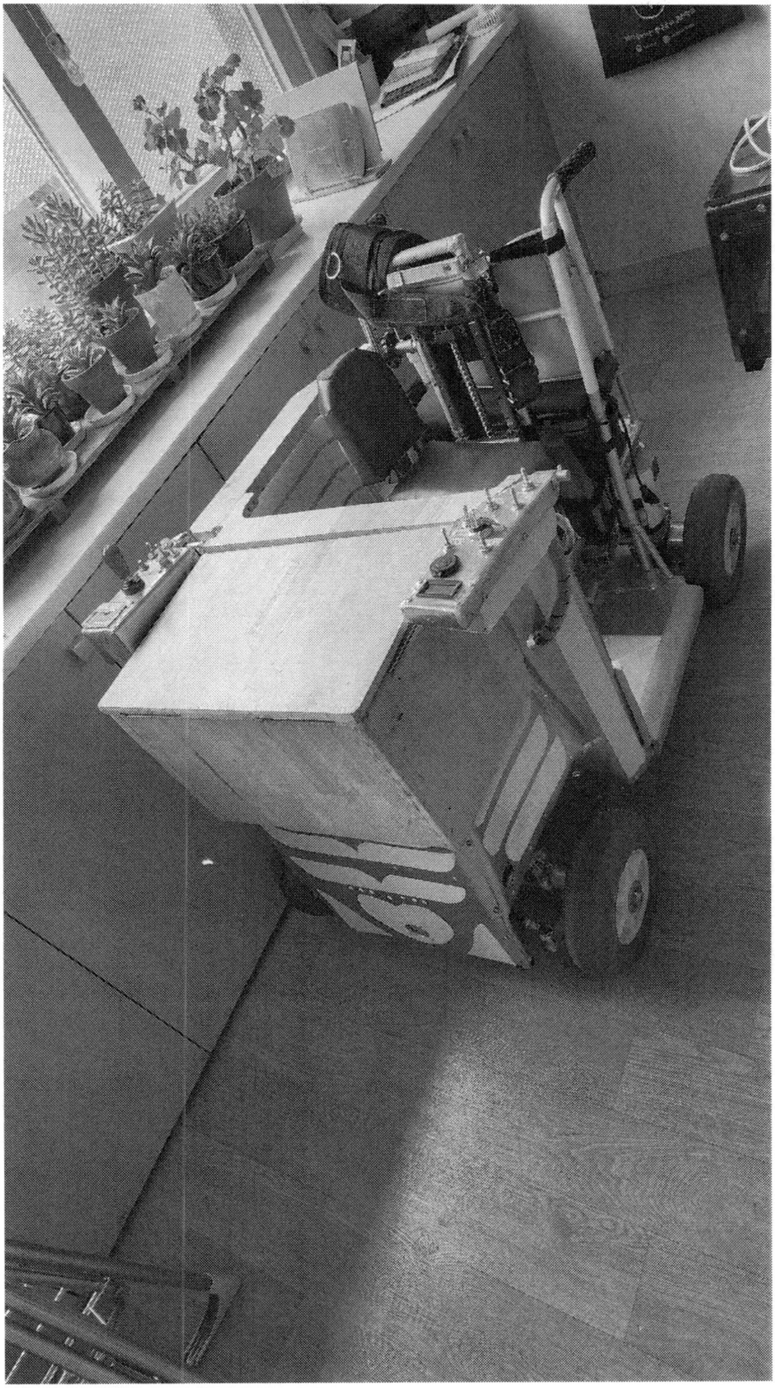

Figure 3.1 Jinju's current motorized wheelchair

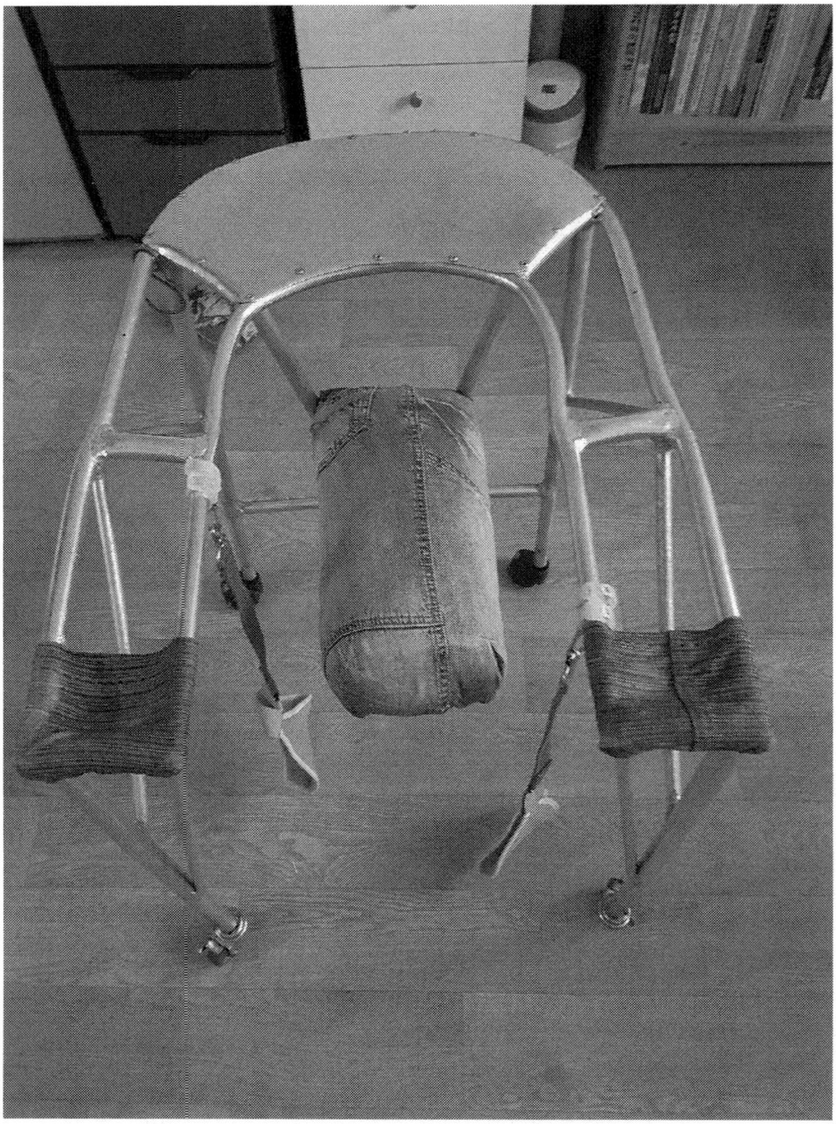

Figure 3.2 Jinju's non-motorized wheelchair designed for indoor use

In middle school, as she continued to grow, her parents struggled to carry her everywhere. They thought it was time for her to use a wheelchair and started contacting wheelchair companies and manufacturers because she could only sit on seats in the shape of a bicycle seat or saddle. All of them responded that they could not invest resources and time into making a customized wheelchair only for Jinju. The journey to find the person who ended up making her wheelchair was long and not easy:

> One day, my parents read a news article about a person who made a customized electric wheelchair for a child with congenital limb difference. He made a wheelchair that was operated by pressing a button with the forehead. My parents asked many people to find his contact information and finally got it. When they first contacted him, he rejected the request saying that he made customized wheelchairs because he wanted to help disadvantaged children with severe disabilities who lived in orphanages and were in difficult situations. He also added that he was an inventor, not someone who specialized in wheelchairs. He volunteered to help the child because he recognized that child lived in an orphanage and had no one else to help. Initially he refused because I had both parents and came from an affluent home environment, so he didn't think that I met the criteria he created for needing his help. But to us, he was our only hope, so my parents begged for him to at least just meet me, and we visited him. After seeing me come in on my mother's back and that I could only sit on either my mom's or dad's lap, he saw how much I needed his help and agreed to make me a wheelchair. He realized that no one else was willing to help and agreed to make a wheelchair customized to my needs. That's how I got to meet him.

Jinju elaborated further on how her relationship with this person has continued throughout her life and become meaningful for both of them:

> For me, my wheelchair was for my daily activities, so whenever something was wrong, I would call and tell him, "My wheelchair isn't moving," "One of the wheels fell off," "The battery isn't charging," and such. And whenever I visit him to get it fixed, I update him on all my achievements, like "Thanks to you, I'm going to college," "Thanks to you, I traveled abroad." I can sense he is always happy and proud to hear my achievements. I've been using my wheelchair for about 20 years so it's almost time for me to need a new one. But now that he is older, he tells me he is worried about who will make me a wheelchair when he is gone.

This story shows how one person can play a significant part in the lives of people with disabilities. It is also interesting to observe how Jinju's relationship with her wheelchair is very special. Others may see her wheelchair as a sign of what she cannot do, but her electronic wheelchair opened the door to many possibilities for her.

> I was able to achieve all the things in my life through the support of many people. But if I hadn't met that person, I wouldn't have a wheelchair

customized to my needs and would perhaps still depend on my mother's back for my activities. Through the wheelchair, I gained my freedom and an opportunity to become independent. With my wheelchair, I was able to travel and study abroad and dare to shower on my own. It truly made my twenties memorable.

Part III Intersection of her story and my story

Living with the perspective of a nondisabled person in my disabled body

Jinju was the first person I interviewed for this project. It was through serendipities that I was able to build a rapport with her within a relatively short period of time. Several brief email exchanges between two strangers were sufficient to form a meaningful relationship between the researcher and the participant. From the first interview when we talked over Zoom, I realized Jinju and I were able to connect easily and feel comfortable sharing about our lived experiences of disabilities. The experience of interviewing her over Zoom and meeting her in person made me reflect on her experience on a deeper level. I particularly found it interesting how she, the one person with the most physically disabled body in my project, talked about living with the perspective of a nondisabled individual at certain points in her life. Out of all the women in this book, Jinju's physical disability was the most severe, and she needed the most support to go through her daily routine.

Jinju attended only mainstream schools with nondisabled peers from elementary to high school. It was not until her college years that she found opportunities to socialize with other individuals with disabilities and study with them. She shared her process of discovering her own bias and assumptions toward other people with disabilities during college:

> All throughout my school years from kindergarten to high school, I was the only person with disabilities and went to schools with peers without disabilities. It was during college when I met peers with disabilities at school for the first time. When I interacted with the peers with disabilities, I realized my own lack of awareness and sensitivity toward people with disabilities. I made certain mistakes during my first year of college.
>
> There was a period in my life when I had certain preconceptions toward people with disabilities because I was only looking at things from the perspective of a nondisabled person. For example, even though I understood people with disabilities and nondisabled people have different perspectives, I was leaning more toward the thought that people with disabilities need to try harder to socially integrate in larger society. I thought people with disabilities did not make enough effort to try to really understand the perspectives of people without disabilities and just complained about not feeling included. Even if there is a stigma in society for people with disabilities, not trying is in a way accepting the

> stigma. Therefore, people with disabilities need to try harder to break the stigma instead of waiting for nondisabled people to get rid of their biases on their own.

As I reflected on what Jinju said, I thought about how I had been living from the perspective of a nondisabled person. Her ability to reflect on her own biases and assumptions and attempt to challenge her own thinking was refreshing and insightful, and I was challenged to examine my own assumptions. Her reflection process challenged me to reexamine my own experiences and expand my own thinking. My educational experiences except elementary school involved mainstream schools along with nondisabled peers. During most of my adult life, my professional and personal network has not included any close connections with individuals with visible disabilities. Therefore, all of my friends except one person are nondisabled. It is interesting to notice how easy it is for me to forget that I have a disability when I hang around my nondisabled friends. I realized how I had my own biases toward other people with disabilities. If an individual with severe physical disabilities, like Jinju, is able to problematize her own thinking toward others with disabilities, how important is it for all of us, regardless of disabilities, to reflect on and challenge our own assumptions?

A unique issue emerged from Jinju's story: the role of spirituality in the lived experience of disability

Jinju is a Christian, and her faith is very important in her personal and professional life. During the interviews, Jinju first shared with me her identity as a Christian. This was very clear when she talked about the vision in her life, and her faith was a critical part of her identity and life mission:

> When I started my undergraduate program, I chose my major in social welfare and decided to work in this field. As a person with disabilities, I feel I am called to take on a meaningful role in contributing to the advocacy work for individuals with disabilities. I believe this was God's plan that I was born with disabilities and sent to this world with a special calling. I realize God has led me through a special life journey. I noticed that church communities need to be more aware and educated about people with disabilities, and I would like to work with churches in this endeavor. After I did my talk for one of the disability awareness events, pastors from several churches saw my talk on YouTube and reached out to ask me if I could give a personal testimony at their churches. I was able to visit two or three churches to share the testimony as well as the lecture on disability awareness before the COVID pandemic. If I am given more opportunities, I'd like to visit more churches and share my testimony of what God has done through me and how He has shown me His love and grace throughout my life. That is one of my visions and dreams.

When I asked Jinju about her role as a disability advocate, she used the metaphor of a bridge and said her career was closely connected to her lived experience as a disabled individual as well as deeply rooted in her Christian faith:

> I see my role as a "bridge" between what may seem like two different worlds – people with disabilities and nondisabled people. Even though I can see how nondisabled people may think of people with disabilities in general, I, as a person with disabilities, am biased and can understand better the perspectives of people with disabilities. I would like to play a role in society to reduce the extent of discrimination against disabilities and support people with disabilities to find what they can do best. I think lack of communication and knowledge, plain ignorance, and misunderstanding can lead to different points of views [between people with disabilities and nondisabled people]. I feel that God has given me this unique role of being a bridge, and this has become part of my identity. I clearly recognize the importance of this calling and remind myself of this calling many times.

When Jinju shared how her Christian faith is connected to the purpose in her life, I was able to empathize with her and connect to her in a unique way because I am also serious about my faith. As a Christian, I believe my disability is a gift from God, enriching my life on this earth. We both have a strong identity as Christians, and our faith plays an important role in the meaning-making process of our lived experiences. For her, faith is a crucial element in shaping the meaning associated with her disability, contributing to a positive perspective. Reflecting on the influence of faith as a Christian, I find little reservations about including this aspect in the book. There's a certain discomfort, as it might not align with the perceived political correctness of discussing religion in academically oriented publications. When talking about the lived experience of disability, factors such as race, gender, culture, and sexuality are brought into conversation as intersectionality, but religion and faith are rarely mentioned. Jinju's story illustrates how the disability experience is woven through multiple identifiers, including religion and faith. It becomes imperative to emphasize the role of Christianity in shaping the experiences of individuals with disabilities, particularly in finding purpose and meaning in life.

4 Theresa

Questioning moments of marginalization and moving beyond barriers

> 저는 고등학교3학년까지는 특수학교만 다녔던 거잖아요. 그러니까 장애인들 속에서는 어떻게 지내야 하는지 어떻게 다가가야 하는지, 이런 것들을 너무나 잘 알고 있는데, 특수학교만 다니다가 대학교에 딱 들어갔을 때, 처음에 비장애학생들하고 친해지고 이렇게 다가가고 하는 것에 있어서 되게 어렵더라고요. 힘들고 . . . 혹시나 내가 그냥 나는 편하게 이야기한 건데 저 친구가 오해하면 어떻게 하지? 막 이런 생각들도 되게 많았고, 그러다 보니까 특수학교에 다니더라도 비장애인들하고 이렇게 많이 부딪힐 수 있는 시간들이 조금 더 많았으면 좋겠다 라는 생각은 들더라고요.
>
> [I only went to special education school until I attended university. So I know very well how to approach and get along with peers with disabilities. But when I went to university after only attending special education school, it was difficult for me to approach nondisabled peers at first and build relationships with them. It was tough. I wondered what I should do if they misunderstood my intentions when I said something. I've had a lot of thoughts like this. I wish I'd had some more opportunities to interact with able-bodied peers even though I went to special education school.]
>
> – Theresa

Theresa is a 40-year-old woman with cerebral palsy who works as a disability advocate in a local branch of a nonprofit organization. Her job is to manage all aspects of the local branch. She also gives speeches to people and organizations to raise awareness of disability-related issues. Theresa feels satisfied and finds meaning in her job: "It is something I'm very good at and I enjoy doing. I also get to meet many people and have a great time, giving me energy."

Theresa was born and raised in South Korea. She is the oldest child in a two-parent household and has one younger brother, who is married and has a child. At the time I interviewed her for this project, she was living alone in a city three hours from Seoul. It was natural for Theresa to get her own place when her parents moved to the countryside, and she needed to live near her workplace for an easier commute. Her parents' home is a 30-minute car ride from her place. Her brother and his family live in the next town over, so she can easily reach his family in case of an emergency.

DOI: 10.4324/9781003609179-4

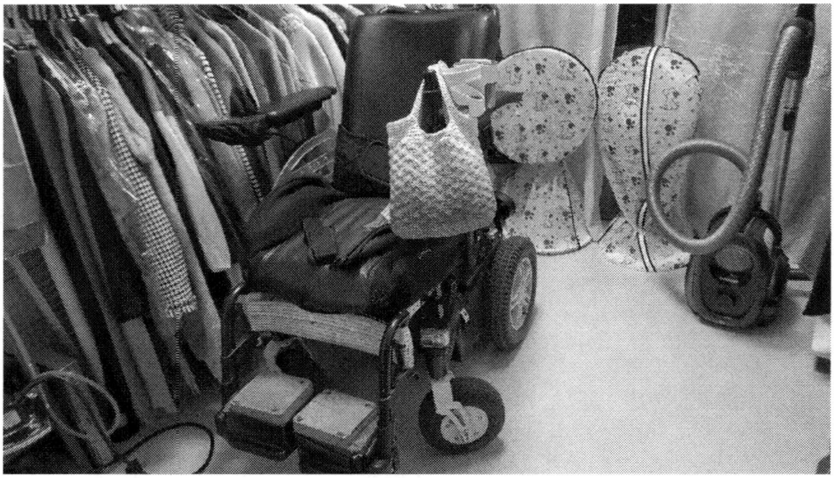

Figure 4.1 Theresa's customized electric wheelchair

Theresa has no speech impairment and has not received any speech therapy. She shared with me that she started talking at seven months, and her disability was not detected until much later. She said, "I think they [parents] didn't suspect I had a disability even though I didn't have neck and head control, since I started talking so early." Theresa can walk independently inside her home but uses a wheelchair for mobility outside. She also has muscle spasms in her neck. She started walking at the age of 7, later than the typical developmental milestone, but her walk was not very stable so in the seventh grade, she started using a wheelchair. She used a manual wheelchair when she was younger and switched to an electronic wheelchair as an adult. When I asked her to identify an object that represented who she was, she mentioned her electronic wheelchair (Figure 4.1).

Theresa: The first [representative object] would be my electric wheelchair.
Yoon Joo: Why?
Theresa: Because I wouldn't be able to get around without it . . . [laughing]. It is always a part of me. I've made some personal touches to it by giving it a splash of pink. The common color for wheelchairs is something like black or silver. But I used pink to accentuate it a little bit.
Yoon Joo: Why did you do that?
Theresa: I didn't want the same thing as everyone else [laughing]. I always like to show my individuality and personality through different things, and my wheelchair is one of them. [The logo color] on my YouTube channel is also pink, so I guess that's why I matched it with pink.
Yoon Joo: How long has it been long since you personalized it?

Theresa: It's been one or two years.
Yoon Joo: Is there anything in particular that inspired you to do so?
Theresa: When I was watching a YouTube clip of another individual with disabilities, she changed the color of her wheelchair. When I saw her wheelchair with unique colors, I noticed it left a good impression on me. I started associating the colors with her. So I personalized mine so I could have a lasting impression on others.

It is clear that to Theresa, the wheelchair is not a symbol of deficit but a part of who she is that enables her to accomplish many things. She acknowledges the challenges she faces but at the same celebrates her accomplishments. She also thinks of roses as a symbolic image of her life:

> If you look at roses, they have thorns on their stems, but at the end of the stems, the flowers blossom so beautifully. There were so many obstacles that I encountered in my life, a lot of things that I thought I couldn't do. But when I reflect on those things as time goes by, I realize there have been more things I was able to achieve. So, I feel like a rose is symbolic of my life.

Theresa receives services from a disability support worker for 20 hours a week on weekdays. In Korea, disability support workers provide care services for people with disabilities who have challenges in daily functioning. If they are eligible for services, disability support workers visit their homes to assist them in their daily lives and help them live independently. Theresa tries to do many housekeeping chores by herself but receives help from the disability support worker in cleaning her place and preparing meals, especially when her physical condition is not well. As Theresa has gotten older, she has developed arthritis in her neck due to her spastic condition, and it is becoming harder to take care of herself. The disability support worker also accompanies Theresa when she goes to places that are not physically accessible.

Part I Encountering: "to come upon face to face"

Connecting with Theresa through Jinju

I was introduced to Theresa by Jinju. They attended the same university and majored in social welfare. In college, they spent a lot of time together since they lived in the dorms, and they have had similar career path as disability advocates. When I interviewed Jinju, she shared several stories about Theresa, and I was very intrigued when she talked about how Theresa's perspective on disability was different from her own viewpoint. Jinju commented that Theresa dealt with certain situations differently and thought this was because their schooling experiences had been different. I told Jinju that I wanted to invite Theresa for an interview and asked her to introduce me to her.

When I invited Theresa to participate in this project, she was happy and willing to share her experience. I had a strong impression that Jinju and Theresa's friendship was very special. Just as Jinju considered Theresa her very close friend, Theresa thought of Jinju as a very close friend, too. When I asked Theresa to identify individuals besides her family members who have made a significant impact on her life, she mentioned Jinju and said the following:

> Jinju and I have been friends since we were 20 years old. I actually spoke to her on the phone before we started our interview. Since we are on very similar career paths, we can often share our ideas and rely on each other for support and encouragement. She takes up a huge part of my life along [laughing]. We live in different provinces, so we can't see each other often. But both Jinju and I are part of the same disability advocacy organization. I started first, then Jinju joined the Seoul location about a year later. She is working for the main center, and I'm working for a local branch.

While Jinju had attended only mainstream schools, Theresa had attended segregated special education settings from elementary to high school. After interviewing both of them, I realized how significantly school settings could affect lived experiences of disability. Especially since Theresa did not live in Seoul, her experiences were somewhat different from those of the other women in this project. I had not thought deeply about differences in access to school choices and the extent of special education services because I had only lived in Seoul and had taken for granted access to mainstream settings. Not only are choices in schools and services different, but general perceptions and responses toward people with disabilities are also different in smaller cities compared to in Seoul. Theresa shared many stories of how she was perceived negatively, marginalized, and denied opportunities because of her visible disabilities.

Childhood memories of marginalization and exclusion

Living in a rural area, Theresa experienced limited access to and opportunities for inclusive education and special education services that were appropriately suited to meet her needs. She described her options for school:

> There weren't any elementary schools for students with physical disabilities near where I lived, so I had to attend a special school for intellectual disabilities for elementary school. The elementary special education school that I attended didn't have curriculum and services that were most appropriate for my levels. So, starting from middle school, I went to a special education school for students with physical disabilities located in Asan in Gyeonggi Province, outside the city where I lived. It was one of the largest special education schools [in Korea].

> This school was both an educational setting and rehabilitation center. There are two classes per grade for the middle and high schools. I lived close to my elementary school, but starting from middle school, I had to stay in the dorms since it was all the way in Gyeonggi.

As Theresa described her educational experiences, she talked about her childhood wish to be in a mainstream setting:

Theresa: I always wanted to attend mainstream schools, but I wasn't allowed to. I resented and hated the fact that there weren't any other school options.

Yoon Joo: Why did you want to attend a mainstream school?

Theresa: I still have the same thought as an adult. I've always thought that I should do the same things as nondisabled people. It wasn't that I couldn't accept my disability. I just couldn't understand why people with disabilities had to be segregated into a separate school. Why couldn't we just attend the same school?

Yoon Joo: Wow, you had very forward thinking, even as a young child. Could you elaborate on what you were thinking back then?

Theresa: Now I think about it. . . . I didn't want to admit that I was different from nondisabled people. I know I had to but didn't want to admit it. I wanted to do the same things as nondisabled people. Since I had this strong desire, I think I was a little depressed throughout childhood. Because I attended special education schools with only peers with disabilities, I had no opportunities to meet and interact with nondisabled peers. That's why I had those feelings. I felt like I was always missing a part of my school experience.

Yoon Joo: Reflecting on what you felt then, how do you feel about it now?

Theresa: Was it because I was a little immature? [laughing]

Yoon Joo: Immature? In what aspect?

Theresa: Wouldn't it have been better if I had just accepted the difference and focused on getting along better with my friends at the [special education] schools?

Yoon Joo: But listening to your happiest childhood memory [shared earlier in the interview], it sounds like you had a wonderful time with your friends [at the special education schools]. After all, you had those friends who decided to make that rebellious escape with you, right?

Theresa: [laughing] That's true.

I was surprised to hear that Theresa, from a very young age, noticed the limited access to opportunities because of her disability and had longings to be included with nondisabled peers. I didn't recall any moment when I really wanted to experience inclusion settings at a very young age. I was very happy to attend a special education elementary school for six years. I remember my disabled body was different from others but did not necessarily think about the importance of taking part in the mainstream world. Maybe my desire for inclusion had not been as strong because I began attending mainstream settings in middle school. I wonder if I would have felt the same way as Theresa if I had not had access to mainstream settings. I didn't question why I was perceived differently, unlike Theresa, who vividly noticed her difference.

At the same time, as I think back on Theresa's comment, it feels uncomfortable and unsettling that she saw herself as "immature" when she was questioning why her presence was denied and excluded from inclusion. It seemed like she had accepted the widespread Korean view that she was different, and it was natural for her to accept the limited access. When I asked Theresa what she thought of this and what she had thought as a child, she answered:

> Since I was a child, I was exposed to many incidences of discrimination because I had a [visible] disability. So I wonder whether I was able to discern that things were not supposed to be like that even though I was just a kid.

As a follow-up, I asked whether she remembered other specific childhood experiences of being discriminated against, and she shared the following incident:

> Even though I was attending a special education school, my mom sent me to a hagwon [private educational institute] so that I would be on track with the general education curriculum. I also told my mom that I wanted to go to a hagwon. So my mom sent me to the hagwon for learning English that my brother was also attending. I attended one session for a day, and then I couldn't go there anymore. The parents of the other students complained about having a child with disabilities in the same class as their children. So I went to the hagwon for a day and wasn't allowed to return. I would have been able to understand the perspectives of these parents if I couldn't keep up with the class material, but on that day, when the teacher asked me questions, I was able to answer the teacher in English. But just because I had a disability, the parents made a complaint, and I never set foot in that hagwon again.

Theresa explained further that at that time, her mom had initially looked into enrolling her at a mainstream elementary school. But all the schools in her neighborhood gave excuses, such as there were too many stairs in the building, no accessible bathrooms, and no ramps. That was how she ended up at a special education school. Unlike the other women in this book, Theresa attended only special education schools until college. Her story illustrates how access to inclusive education can vary depending on local contexts even in a relatively small country like Korea. It is not appropriate to assume that lived experiences of disability are the same, even within the same country. Theresa's own words highlight this point:

> Since I am from a rural area, my experience may seem a bit extreme and cannot be generalized. However, I don't think the characteristics of the rural context can be ignored.

Part II Embracing: "accept or support willingly and enthusiastically"

Taking charge and advocating for herself

I found Theresa to be a forward-thinker and a strong advocate for herself because she has tried many things that I did not think about even for myself. For example, I discovered that she is a sprinter. She talked about the importance of physical training in her life as an adult:

> I'm a thrower in a wheelchair. I feel obligated to exercise. Even though I don't practice very hard, I basically keep going to strengthen my muscles. I have always been a part of a [sports] program to do so. I am being trained at a gym for people with disabilities in the city where I live, Guri. The gym has training programs that are in accordance with my needs. This physical exercise is beneficial. As an adult, I haven't been receiving any physical therapy, so I have been able to maintain my current physical health for a longer period of time because of this physical training.

Theresa started becoming involved in sports while attending special education school. She did not receive physical therapy when she was a child, but in school, there were always designated times for physical education. She and her peers had the opportunity to explore different types of adaptive physical activities or sports, such as boccia, which made it more likely for her to join parasports later on:

Yoon Joo: Was PE class very different in your school since it was only for students with disabilities?
Theresa: Yes . . . . We had many opportunities to play sports, like boccia and such.
Yoon Joo: What was your favorite thing about PE?
Theresa: Me? I didn't really like PE [laughing]. The teachers encouraged me to be an athlete, but I didn't start [athletic training] until I was in my 20s. I'm still competing.
Yoon Joo: Are you playing sports in your wheelchair?
Theresa: Yes, I'm a thrower.

Yoon Joo: Ah, you must be very active.
Theresa: I started it without thinking too much about it, but the coach wouldn't let me quit.
Yoon Joo: You must've been good for the coach to do that.
Theresa: Probably because I'm still capable of getting a medal. I'm participating in the national sports competition this year too.
Yoon Joo: How many times have you participated in the competition?
Theresa: I've been an athlete for about 13 years, so it's my 13th time so far competing. I compete in throwing in the field. This is one of the sports for people with cerebral palsy, and this game is about throwing a long distance.
Yoon Joo: Wow, that sounds amazing. I wish more people could find out about this [sports competitions for people with disabilities].
Theresa: You're right. Even many people with disabilities aren't familiar with the different sports [that people with disabilities can play].
Yoon Joo: As an individual with disabilities, I didn't know about this. This is really unexpected. It's amazing how active you are.

Before the interviews, I had no idea that Theresa was an athlete competing in the Paralympic Games in Korea. Even though I knew about these competitions, I did not expect to meet an athlete while conducting this project. Also, I might have assumed that Theresa was too old to play in a national sports competition. As I recall Theresa's story, I realize how stuck I was in my own assumptions and biases on age and disability within the context of sports.

Theresa was also proactive in figuring out solutions when faced with challenges. In college, she had not studied very hard, and her GPA was not good enough to qualify for a scholarship. She really needed a scholarship to continue her college education since her family was not financially well-off. This was how she dealt with the situation:

> There was a support center for students with disabilities in the university I attended, and those who worked as aids at this center received scholarships. So I went to the center blindly and said to the center director, "I'd like to apply for an aid position." At first, the center director was speechless and confused because I, a disabled student who was more likely to be a recipient of help, was asking to be a helper. But I repeatedly begged the director, explaining that I really needed money to continue my studies. I told him, "I may not be able to attend the university if I don't get a scholarship." Finally, the director gave in and told me to be a mobility assistant [moving to and from lecture halls] for students with visual impairments. So, I was able to get a scholarship.

To earn money for her tuition, Theresa was forced to step up, and this challenging situation served as a catalyst that changed her own mindset. Theresa didn't question her eligibility or capacity to help others with disabilities.

I wonder if this may be due to the fact that she had only attended special education schools prior to college. If she had attended mainstream settings, she might have only experienced situations in which she was in the position of someone who needed help from others. Theresa was not afraid or timid in seeking out opportunities to enrich her studies:

> In my department, able-bodied students did a lot of internships and other practicums [as part of their undergraduate study]. I wanted to do the same thing, too, so I chased after the professors and begged them [for internship opportunities] [laughing]. I begged, "Please let me do this." When I was studying social welfare, I thought that it was important to do a lot of internships. I believed that if I didn't do internships at that time, I would be disadvantaged again when looking for employment later on. To fight against discrimination, I thought the only solution was to demonstrate my capability and competency through internship experiences.

These stories clearly illustrate Theresa's strong sense of agency and how she continually seeks out opportunities to assert her presence even when faced with barriers and limited access at first. When I applauded her proactive attitude, she responded:

> I'm not really the quiet type. I don't think I can sit in an office and do desk work quietly. I have to go out and meet people. I think that's more my tendency.

She also commented, "It's because I'm stupid [laughing]. I'm recklessly brave so I wasn't afraid of trying new things." I found it interesting that Theresa used words such as *meongcheong* (멍청), *yamjeon* (얌전), and *josin* (조신) when describing her attitude in these situations. Her choice of these words makes me wonder if individuals with disabilities are given subtle messages that it is not appropriate to challenge the status quo and the limitations imposed upon them. In particular, she used two adjectives that are usually used to describe women with great virtue in a traditional sense: *Josinhada* translates to being modest and cautious, and *yamjeonhada* means being meek, quiet, and gentle. Theresa described herself as not following the traditional female gender role by just asserting her rights and seeking access when facing barriers and challenges. It is most likely that disabled women in Korea receive subtle, yet clear, messages that they are not supposed to assert their rights too strongly.

Developing social networks with able-bodied peers and mentoring students with disabilities

Theresa talked about her social networks with able-bodied peers as well as students with disabilities. Her college years were when Theresa first experienced real relationships with nondisabled peers. Since she had had no opportunity for meaningful social inclusion in her early years, she was initially very anxious about her peers' perceptions:

Yoon Joo: You shared earlier in the interview that you really wished for more opportunities to share experiences with nondisabled peers. In retrospect, do you think you were able to do so in college?

Theresa: Yes. I feel like I socialized more with able-bodied peers than those with disabilities. But I remember thinking at that time that it would've been easier to socialize with these peers if I'd had the opportunity to attend mainstream schools and been exposed to them sooner.

Yoon Joo: What made you think that?

Theresa: Back then, I was very cautious when approaching nondisabled peers. A part of me was afraid of what they would think when I approached them. I often asked myself. . . . "Would they just think of me as someone who needed their help instead of their friend?"

Yoon Joo: Have those thoughts changed?

Theresa: Yes. Now I socialize well with nondisabled people. I think I am involved in different activities in the community and meet-up groups.

Yoon Joo: Was there a specific moment that helped you overcome your hesitation?

Theresa: During my college years, I had a close guy friend who helped me a lot throughout college. Back then, there were no low-floor buses. But he helped me load the wheelchair on the bus. We would go to watch movies and do other fun activities. I feel like he helped me change my perspective. That's when I realized I just needed to approach them [nondisabled peers] without being so conscious about what I did or who I was.

Yoon Joo: He is such a wonderful friend.

Theresa's time in college was an important milestone for her in truly integrating into mainstream society. Through meaningful friendships, she was able to break her assumptions and biases regarding others' perceptions.

Because she feels she missed out on many opportunities for inclusion earlier in her life and had to seriously advocate for herself to get to where she is now, Theresa is eager to empower other individuals with disabilities so they can be successfully integrated. Since she attended special education schools for many years and has been involved in sports competitions for people with disabilities, she has a wide social network of individuals with disabilities. At the time of the interviews, Theresa was mentoring about 2–3 people whom she had met through acquaintances. She talked about the meaning of mentoring in her life:

> Mentoring gives me the motivation to live my life as best as I can so that I can set a good example for others. Because I am mentoring others,

> I also try to live my life to its fullest potential. Through my mentoring relationship with them, I see that their lives are changed, and it's very rewarding for me to witness changes in their lives. It is hard but necessary. I am thankful that I am able to mentor those who need it as well as others who find it necessary. If I can support or guide in any aspect of their lives, I would like to cultivate mentoring relationships with them.

Theresa shared one specific anecdote from her mentoring experience:

> I'm mentoring a college student right now. Until his second year of high school, he was like, "Theresa, I'm not going to college." I asked, "Why don't you want to go?" and he said, "I am not a good student and don't think I'll be able to get into college." I asked, "What are you going to do if you don't go to college?" He said, "Uh . . . I don't know." He had no plan! So, I spent a year trying to convince him to go to college. He's a really smart kid and should attend a school-like [mainstream] school. But back then, even his parents wanted to send him to a community college nearby because they were afraid of not being able to take care of him if he was far from home. That's why I nagged his mother so much [laughing]. In the end, his mother and I saw eye to eye, and he got into the 4-year senior college in Daegu last year. He was in school, but during the COVID pandemic, classes were remote, and he had to study from home. Soon after, the mom had him take a leave of absence. When I asked him for the reason, he explained that his mom didn't think it was worth attending a university far from home if he was just attending online classes at home and did not have opportunities to socialize with other students. I disagreed with this because the main purpose of college education is in fact studying. I told him, "Do you attend the university to have fun?" I explained that if he delayed a year, it was going to be harder for him and that it was important for him to stay on track. Thankfully, he went back to school this year [laughing].

I admire Theresa's passion and eagerness to guide and advocate for other students with disabilities. At the same time, I was surprised to hear how Theresa encountered those who were not open to her advice and did not take it well when she reached out to challenge them to step out of their comfort zones. She said with a laugh, "My advice is valuable to those who consider my challenge [to advance further] important, but I'm a nuisance to those who don't." I expected that Theresa's willingness to advocate for others would always be welcomed with open arms, but that was not the case. Even though some may not respond positively to Theresa's help, she is adamant about encouraging others with disabilities to challenge the status quo and push themselves above the limit:

> Even now, when I meet other people with disabilities, especially those in their 20s, I often say "Whether it works or not, just try it." [Smiling.] I often say to them, "You need to try it first to truly find out if you can

> do it or not. If you just assume that you can do nothing, you will not be able to accomplish anything, so you need to try even if you do fail. Also, even if you do fail, there's no reason to be disappointed and frustrated. You just need to find other ways, so you need to keep trying." I tend to talk a lot about that.

Theresa's relationships with others illustrate how she embraces her disability identity and continuously strives to self-advocate and to empower others.

Part III Intersection of her story and my story

Empowered through self-contained education settings

I realize that Theresa and I lived such different lives. Honestly, out of all the four women I interviewed, it was most difficult for me to identify shared experiences in Theresa's story. One shared experience I found was that we both attended special education elementary schools. Theresa's story illustrates the pros and cons of attending special education schools with other students with disabilities. Her interview made me reflect on my own experience of attending a special education school and reevaluate the meaning of segregated settings. When talking about special education schools, Theresa voiced concerns about "the missing piece" when she talked about not feeling academically ready for college and having to study extra hard while preparing for the college entrance exam:

> Although special schools used the same curriculum as regular schools, the process was different in certain aspects, such as the pace of the curriculum. Such discrepancies were evident when comparing scores from standardized tests and college entrance exams. Students who attended special schools tended to receive lower scores. I always wished for certain solutions that would narrow the gap in academic programs between these schools.

At the same time, Theresa was able to articulate unique benefits of attending special education schools:

> I think special education schools are important. In special education schools, there are times for other academic subjects as well as times for physical exercise and therapy that are accommodated depending on the characteristics of physical disabilities.

Both academic and social experiences are important components when talking about schooling. Theresa's story reminded me of the powerful impact of a close-knit network with other students with disabilities. Even though it was only six years of elementary school, reflecting back, I remember these years as happy memories and don't recall any distinct "encounter" with my disability. Since all of my elementary school friends had physical disabilities, I felt "normal" and accepted as who I was. I participated in all different types of activities, learning piano and calligraphy, which were taught by volunteers from nearby universities. During PE classes, I often ran around with my peers on the school playground, playing many games. One of our favorite games was Red Light, Green Light. Many times, I helped peers who had more significant physical challenges to get ready for each class by taking out notebooks from their school bags and pushing their wheelchairs around to different parts of the school.

Even though Theresa had wanted to attend mainstream schools, she had good experiences while attending special education schools. She shared a wonderful memory with her friends from high school:

> My happiest memory of high school is being rebellious with my friends. [One evening] we told the teachers that we were going home and got an overnight pass to make a trip to downtown Seoul. Four friends and I took a subway to downtown Seoul and hung out all night at Marronnier Park. At that time, I was in a manual wheelchair, so two of my friends with mild physical disabilities who could walk, pushed my wheelchair whenever we went out. We watched dancers perform and people playing basketball on the street. When it got too cold, we warmed ourselves up by eating ramen at the food court. Then we took the first subway in the morning and returned back to the dorm.

In special education environments, Theresa and I were not perceived as different, disabled, or helpless. I believe that special education environments can be beneficial and empowering because it is less likely for students with disabilities to be marginalized and positioned as powerless. Eventually individuals with disabilities need to be integrated into mainstream society as adults, so it is not appropriate for them to be placed in segregated settings for their entire school experiences. However, the unique and indelible benefits of special education settings need to be acknowledged and highlighted.

A unique issue emerged from Theresa's story: rethinking smiles on my face

Theresa's story made me think about issues that I had not paid serious attention. For example, I did not really have strong yearnings to attend mainstream school since I only attended special education school for six years of my schooling experience. I was very surprised to hear that Theresa had wanted to go to schools with other nondisabled peers. To a certain extent, I was not comfortable with listening to how much she had wanted to go to a mainstream setting because, at first, I felt like she did not appreciate the value of her experiences in special education school. But as she shared her stories about mentoring others with disabilities and her career as a disability advocate, I realized it was not about her feeling resentful about all her years at special education schools but about advocating for her right to be educated as much as possible along nondisabled peers. As I thought back on Theresa's recollection, I learned how essential it is to provide different choices of schools to students with disabilities so they do not feel limited in their schooling experiences.

Theresa's educational experiences in special education school significantly affected how she felt about developing relationships with nondisabled peers. She shared how she was nervous when interacting with them and did not know how to behave. When I first attended mainstream middle school, I went through a similar process. During the first year, I was nervous about initiating friendships with peers and self-conscious about what they thought of me. At lunchtime, I felt awkward eating with them at the same table because I often spilled food while I was eating. I was hyperaware of the abnormality of my disabled body. Theresa did not share detailed stories about making friends with nondisabled peers but clearly articulated her anxiety and concern about socializing with them after attending special education school through high school. She also mentioned how having a smile on her face was important to make her approachable to others:

Theresa: People remember me as someone who smiles a lot. I usually smile a lot. I've heard a lot of people say that it is nice to see me smile so brightly. So I thought about the word "smile" to represent who I am.

Yoon Joo: I see. You must have a very cheerful personality.

Theresa: I try to be.

Yoon Joo: You shared that many people tell you that you smile a lot. Would you agree?

Theresa: I don't do it a lot when I'm by myself. But I tend to smile often when I'm around others. Smiling has become a habit, and now I think I automatically smile when I'm just around people.

Yoon Joo: You said that you tend to laugh a lot when you are around people. Could you elaborate on that a little bit?

Theresa: Ever since I was a child, I have been told many times, "Since you are physically disabled, it will be harder for people to approach you, and you will have a hard time living alongside others if your face is stoic and dark." My mom also told me the same thing several times. That's why I feel pressured to smile a lot so that I can look approachable to other people. To a certain extent, I have learned to keep smiling.

Yoon Joo: Being "pressured"? In a way, doesn't that give a negative connotation? What do you think?

Theresa: When I was young, there were times when it was difficult for me to always smile. Thinking back on those times, it feels unpleasant. Being pressured might sound negative to some people, but it may not be. I believe it could simply be a way of expressing myself.

To a certain extent, I can empathize with Theresa because I have heard often that I have a bright smile. I think I am a pretty positive person, but Theresa's comment brought back memories of hearing similar messages from my parents and others. This is uncomfortable to think about, but I wonder about the things disabled individuals have to do to survive in mainstream society. Because our disabled bodies are often perceived unfavorably and negatively, we are unconsciously compelled to put smiles on our faces to make ourselves presentable and approachable. Disabled individuals are often socialized to camouflage abnormal parts of their bodies with pleasant smiles to integrate with "normal" people.

5 Helen

Living in two countries, South Korea and the United States

> 저는 밤에 잘 때 꿈에서라도 말 잘 하는 꿈을 꾸고 싶은데, 꿈에서도 말이 잘 안 나오는 꿈을 꾸지 꿈에서도 장애가 있는 사람이더라구요.
>
> [I often wish to be able to speak without impairment in my dreams but unfortunately I still have my disability even in my dreams.]
>
> – Helen

Helen is a 52-year-old Korean American woman with cerebral palsy, living in the United States and working as a professor who teaches special education classes at a university located on the East Coast. She is fluent in both English and Korean, and her area of expertise is assistive technology. When I started this project, I wanted to recruit a Korean American woman with visible disabilities living in the United States. A few years ago, I read about Helen in several online articles and watched YouTube clips featuring her and her mother. From the articles, I discovered that when she was 3 years old, she attended the same rehabilitation center for children with orthopedic impairments and physical disabilities that I had attended for elementary school. During our first interview, she told me that she used to stay at the rehabilitation center during the week to receive intensive therapy and come home during the weekend.

Helen grew up as the middle child of three, with one older brother and one younger brother, in a two-parent household. When asked to describe her parents, she said, "My parents have been supportive throughout my entire life, making sure I find happiness in every moment." She attended mainstream elementary, middle, and high schools in Korea and came to the United States to further her studies. She described her study abroad journey as "a bit of a coincidence." She had not been accepted to universities in Korea at the end of her senior year in high school, so she had contemplated spending the following year studying for the college entrance exam and reapplying for college in Korea. At that time, her father asked her if she wanted to study abroad. This was an unexpected option for her, but she said to herself, "Why not?" and decided to go to the United States.

DOI: 10.4324/9781003609179-5

Helen came from an upper-middle-class family background, and her father was able to provide her with financial support to study abroad. Her aunt lived on the East Coast, so she chose to attend the English Language Institute (ELI) there. Her original plan was to return to Korea with her family after completing a bachelor's degree and possibly a graduate degree. But life brought an unexpected turn. She met her husband, who is also Korean American, fell in love, and got married. Helen ended up staying in the United States and received a bachelor's and master's degree in computer science. As she was looking for jobs, she became pregnant with her first child, so she put her job search on hold. Her journey of obtaining a doctorate degree in assistive technology started with her own personal desire to become an accomplished mother to her future children. She and her husband now have two children, a 26-year-old son and a 22-year-old daughter.

While searching online, Helen discovered an assistive technology program at the university where she had completed her bachelor's degree. The term "assistive technology" was initially unfamiliar to her since it was still very new at that time. Seven months after having her first child, she decided to take a course in an extended program to find out about the field. By the end of the course, she was mesmerized by the idea and applied it to the master's program in assistive technology. In the following semester when she began her studies, she was fortunate to meet her advisor, who was a pioneer in the field. He suggested Helen pursue the PhD program. Helen successfully completed her doctorate degree and received from her advisor an offer to teach assistive technology in the same program that she had completed for her doctorate study. She has been teaching at this university for more than 15 years.

Part I Encountering: "to come upon face to face"

Sharing many similar life experiences

Before I interviewed Helen for this project, we had never met, but we were able to connect quickly during the first interview as we started talking about teachers we knew in common from the rehabilitation center. We also shared many similar experiences. During the second interview when I asked her whether she had any particular thoughts after the first interview, she commented, "As I responded to the interview questions, you also shared some of your experiences. Listening to your experiences and hearing how similar they were to mine helped me feel a connection with you."

Throughout the three interviews I conducted with her, I was amazed by how Helen and I had dealt with similar issues in life since we had lived in both Korea and the United States. I acknowledge that we have been privileged, given many opportunities in the United States compared to our counterparts who live in Korea. Our parents were able to provide financial support for us to study abroad. To many individuals with disabilities and their families in

Korea, this is quite a huge privilege because they have the preconceived notion that the United States is a land of opportunity and access, especially for those with disabilities. Helen clearly articulated her advantaged background:

> My dad was an owner of a big company, so I was fortunate to have the option of studying abroad. In the 80s, it wasn't common to study abroad, but my parents were able to financially support me along with all the love they showered me with. I'm always grateful for the support, especially the financial support I had because I see many families who have children with disabilities want to come to America but cannot afford to. I feel like even knowing the hardships of the language barrier and other challenging aspects of living in America, parents are willing to come since they want to provide an education for their disabled children.

By living in two countries, we experienced the impact of different social and cultural contexts on the formation of our disability identity. We are emergent bilinguals whose first language is Korean and who had the experience of being caught in a space where we needed to negotiate between two different cultures. We are very familiar with dealing with cultural and language barriers. Our lived experiences are marked by multiple social identities. Even though we were given many privileges, our lives were not always rosy. As women of color with disabilities living in a foreign land, we certainly experienced marginalization because of our intersectional identities arising from being women, disabled, and a racial minority.

Life in Korea: encountering negative stereotypes due to visible disabilities

Helen attended mainstream elementary, middle, and high schools in Seoul. In the 1980s, very few students with disabilities were allowed to attend a mainstream school along with nondisabled peers. Naturally, Helen faced situations in which others underestimated her abilities because of her physical disability. She shared that her elementary school years were uneventful since she attended a small private school with only three classes per grade. But once in middle school, which had a considerably bigger population, she had to deal with situations in which she stood out as the only student with disabilities. She shared the following story:

> Compared to my elementary school, my middle school had a larger population since students from other cities joined the school. Since I was one of the shorter students, I would always be seated toward the front of the classrooms. During lunch time, peers from other classrooms would come and look at me eat through one of classroom windows like they were watching a monkey in a zoo.

With many classmates, however, Helen witnessed changes in their attitudes and interactions as the school year progressed:

> At first, they [other students] were like, "Who is she?" but once they got to know me, they began to understand me. Slowly peers got to know me as a person. Eventually we established genuine friendships. Overall, my relationships with peers were decent.

It was not only students but also teachers who perceived Helen as different from the rest of the group. Her stories illustrate how the teachers were unable to see beyond her disability. As she reflected on her teachers, she was able to articulate why they reacted in such a way:

> It was interesting for me to observe the teachers' initial responses. These days, a lot of people in South Korea have more exposure and are much more aware of people with disabilities through the media, etc. But at the time, when I was attending middle and high school, many people rarely met people with disabilities and didn't know how to treat them. I think that was why teachers and staff were shocked and surprised to see me in their classrooms. For example, it must have been in middle school. Don't you [Yoon Joo] remember that students in middle schools in Korea always lined up according to height? So on the first day of every school year, all the students lined up in the hallway before going into the classroom. I was the fourth shortest student in the class, so I was the fourth student in the line. When the homeroom teachers came out into the hallway to greet the students in their class for the first time in the school year, I saw how they were shocked and surprised to see me. Something like that happened at the beginning of every school year in middle and high school.

There were other instances when teachers underestimated her ability and showed implicit bias:

> After the fall midterm of my first year of middle school, one of the teachers called out individual students' names and their grades on the exams, one after another. As the teacher announced each student's name in front of the whole class, after calling out my name, there was a puzzled look on the teacher's face, followed by the comment, "Huh, your score is good." It was as if she assumed that my score would be low because of my disability.

During the interviews, Helen shared many positive stories of being successfully integrated into mainstream schools. She made several friends, and these close relationships have continued into her adult life. However, Helen still experienced negative stereotyping and was treated differently. She talked about how she wanted to try many things, but people assumed that she could not do them. She said:

> Even as a child, during gym class, the teachers would tell me to take it easy or simply to not participate at all. But I still participated to the best of my ability. I thought it would help me to try all the things that other friends were doing.

Her life motto has been to give everything a try and seize opportunities, and that is how she usually approaches situations. It was interesting to hear how others communicated the messages of "You are different" and "You cannot do it," but she operated from the mindset of ableism and with a positive attitude:

> Sometimes the teachers thought they were being considerate when they excluded me from physical activities during PE class. But I actually wanted to participate. I wish they'd ask individual students with disabilities [what they want to do] instead of assuming [what they can or cannot do].

Living as a nonnative English speaker with disabilities in the United States

Helen's native language is Korean, and she learned English when she came to the United States after graduating from high school. It takes a long time for many people to become completely fluent in written and spoken English, especially when they come to the United States later in their lives. Because of her cerebral palsy, Helen has minor articulation challenges; however, it is not hard to understand her when she speaks in Korean. The interviews were conducted in Korean, and I had no problem understanding her speech even though it was my first time meeting her. When talking about her life in the United States, Helen mentioned her challenges were related to communication because of her articulation difficulties. This communication issue seems to be more complicated because she is not a native English speaker; she didn't mention her speech when talking about her childhood and adolescent years. Helen faced challenges not only as an individual with speech impairment but also as an English language learner:

> English is forever a working progress for people like us who come to America at a later age. My English pronunciation simply does not work. I can read and write English well. But it is difficult to speak in English. I realized that I would need to practice speaking English in order to improve. But I didn't have many opportunities to, even in ESL class. I'm embarrassed by my level of speaking in English, given the long years I've lived here.

Helen explained that she stayed silent when she was studying computer science, before discovering the field of assistive technology:

> In the past when I didn't know and use AAC [augmentative alternative communication], I kept my mouth shut. My bachelor's and master's degrees were in computer science, so I didn't need to converse much for the courses. It was just listening to lectures, turning in assignments, and taking exams. When I had a question, I would visit the professor and ask so there wasn't much interaction with classmates. I just focused on studying alone during my years in undergraduate and graduate school.

With the help of technology, Helen had easier access to communication in English with others. When she started her doctorate program in assistive technology, she began to use an AAC device:

> About a year after I started my PhD program, I attended an Assistive Technology conference with my professor and there were several types of AAC devices to try. After trying a few, I found one that was compatible with my needs, and I started using it the second year of my PhD.

When Helen changed her fields from computer science to assistive technology, the extent of her participation and opportunities broadened, showing that an individual's experience of disability may change greatly depending upon social contexts and the tools given to them. The AAC device provided many opportunities for Helen to actively participate in different settings. It became an alternative way of using her voice in social contexts, enabling her to thrive personally and professionally. She said, "I usually use my AAC to communicate. I can manage to do small talk without it, but it is very challenging pronouncing certain English words without using my AAC device." Her educational background, successful completion of her doctorate degree, and her career path in academia illustrate her high competency in written English and reading. She has been able to achieve the American dream but still has experienced barriers as a nonnative English speaker with disabilities:

> I felt like a stranger. My speech impairment seemed to be the biggest reason for that, even though I knew that wasn't to blame. America is a country full of opportunities. Even a person like me could be a professor. I wonder . . . if I had completed my PhD in Korea, would my advisor have suggested I pursue teaching in college? Sometimes I wish that I didn't have my speech impairment so that I could take advantage of all the opportunities in America, where there is less stigma toward people with disabilities. It's just wishful thinking since the only inconvenient thing for me living in the U.S. is language-related.

Even though the AAC device has played an important role in Helen's life, limitations still existed:

> When I needed to use my AAC for in-person [faculty] meetings before the pandemic, by the time I was done inputting what I wanted to say, they had moved on to another topic. Unless it was very important, I just disregarded what I was going to share.

Her experience of meetings drastically changed during the COVID pandemic when meetings began to be held online:

> For the past two years since the pandemic began, all the meetings at my university have been online. My participation during meetings has actually increased thanks to the chat feature in Zoom. I suppose that is one benefit the pandemic has provided me. If I made a spelling error in the Zoom chat, it was no big deal because this was a common mistake that other faculty members also had. If I happened to make a spelling error [during in-person meetings], the AAC read it verbatim which could be awkward. Overall, it is much more convenient and easier for me to express my thoughts via chat during meetings.

She explained she has tried to be more proactive during meetings:

> I always request for the captioning option to be turned on for Zoom meetings, so that I don't miss any information. At the beginning of a meeting, I let the participants know that I will be using the chat feature to communicate. I also ask for a designated reader to read my chats out loud for the meeting.

I noticed with interest how empowered Helen felt during these meetings. Before I listened to her experience, I had assumed that many individuals were more likely to be silenced and marginalized during video conferencing, but Helen's experience made me rethink their effectiveness. Helen's story illustrates how one can feel empowered or marginalized by different factors interacting within a specific context. It is not all disability that creates an experience of feeling deficient and marginalized, but how disability is manifested and treated in an environment by other people.

Part II Embracing: "accept or support willingly and enthusiastically"

Empowered by two important mentors

While Helen was attending mainstream schools in Korea, many teachers treated her with bias, often underestimating her social and academic abilities:

> In many classrooms in Korea, students are assigned to specific numbers in the alphabetical order of their names. Then the teachers would call

> out students' numbers to indicate their turn to read an excerpt from a book. Many times, when my number was called, I wouldn't want to read because I didn't feel confident even though I always wanted to do it. Also, most teachers would skip my turn and call the next student.

These teachers did not give Helen opportunities to participate, skipping her turn for activities, such as reading out loud. However, when I asked Helen to identify significant people outside of her family, she mentioned one specific teacher who taught her Korean language arts during her junior year of high school:

> This teacher was different. She called me by my name: "Helen, please try to read the next passage." So I stood up and read it. By the time I was done, I had tears rolling down my face. I'm still not sure why I cried. . . . Was I embarrassed because I didn't read it so well? Or was I grateful to have finally gotten a chance to participate? Later, the teacher wrote me a letter. She wrote, "Never let the fear of how others might judge you take away opportunities from you. You do you." It meant so much to me, and I still have that letter. I also still keep in touch with her.

This teacher gave Helen significant encouragement to be more confident in mainstream settings. Although the other teachers did not fully integrate her in their teaching, one teacher was able to make a positive impact on her life.

Helen also talked a lot about her mentor, the advisor in her doctorate program. Assistive technology has been a major part of Helen's life as she holds a doctorate degree in this area, teaches students about assistive technology, and, most importantly, uses AAC devices in many situations. She said, "My advisor was the one who helped me discover my life career, and I am very grateful for him." She shared how she started teaching at a university:

> I received a doctorate degree in 2004. As I got closer to finishing my dissertation, my advisor asked if I would be interested in teaching students at the college. This question threw me off guard. I don't know how your disability affects you, Yoon Joo, but speaking for myself, I speak better when interacting one-on-one. But when it comes to anything more than that, I get easily nervous, feel stiffer here [pointing to her vocal cords], and cannot speak clearly. So never had I considered teaching others because of my disability. When I shared this with my advisor, he gave me words of encouragement. He said that I had a respectable education background and advised me to utilize an AAC device effectively when teaching others. This gave me the courage to start teaching my first class in the fall of 2004, the same year I graduated.

Even when Helen was doubting her own ability and not confident about her potential, her advisor reassured her so she could take a step of faith. These two teachers made significant impacts and challenged her to rise above the occasion.

Empowering others through her teaching

Her career as a professor in the field of special education holds significant meaning in Helen's life personally and professionally. When I asked her, "What is your life like as a professor?" she said:

> If I had continued pursuing my studies in computer science and become a professor in computer science, I imagine being a professor would have simply been just my occupation. However, since I pursued my PhD in assistive technology and became a professor in the field of special education, my job is closely related to my personal life. Therefore, being a professor seems like an important aspect of my life and my identity as who I am.

Helen found strong satisfaction in helping students break down their own biases toward students with disabilities as they learned from her:

> Most of my students are aspiring special education teachers and various service providers such as physical therapists, occupational therapists, speech and language pathologists, etc. Giving my students hope is the most rewarding feeling. At the time my course was offered in-person, I had a few students who shared their honest opinion that they were surprised to see me as their instructor. But it is a very good feeling when the students share their experiences of implementing what they learned during my class and tell me how helpful the course content was when they worked with children.

In addition, Helen was very proud to share her accomplishment of receiving two teaching awards:

> I felt very honored. I received a teaching award in 2012, then another in 2020. The one in 2020 was an online teaching award. The award I received in 2012 was for in-person teaching. The online teacher awards started in 2018, due to the world we live in now. Students and other faculty members had nominated me, so I had to make a combined portfolio and submit it. The process entailed a lot of work, but I was thrilled to have received the online teacher award in 2020.

The teaching awards are one of the most meaningful achievements for Helen since they show how students in her class acknowledged her merit as a professor:

> It makes me wonder how someone like me, who came to America not knowing much English and is an AAC user, ended up teaching students and moreover receiving a teaching award. It felt surreal to receive the

> award. Receiving the award gave me confidence, and I felt it represented who I wanted to be. I know some other people who receive the award don't care too much about this award. But for me, it was so special and like a dream come true.

Helen's strong passion for teaching and identity as a professor has clearly empowered her and enabled her to empower others:

> When I envision myself in the next 5, 10 years, I hope I am still teaching as a professor and expanding my contributions to the field of assistive technology and AAC. I'd like to put myself forward in the field of AAC and support people who can benefit from using an AAC to communicate. Also, I would like to raise awareness of communication disabilities and educate others on how to communicate with people who use AAC. Currently my focus is teaching but I believe there needs to be more research opportunities related to AAC. Starting last year, I shared how I benefited from our meetings converting to online due to the pandemic. . . . In this way, I would like to slowly expand my influence and input in the next 5 to 10 years.

I completely understand how Helen's career in academia and preparing special education teachers is very meaningful and beyond just a job in her life since I am also in the same position. As a full-time professor, I have been teaching in a graduate special education program for about 20 years. I teach courses on disabilities to graduate students preparing to become special education teachers. Throughout my career in academia, my personal experiences as someone with a physical disability have been integrated into my teaching. In classes, when discussing certain issues, such as social inclusion, challenges for people with disabilities across their life span, and assumptions about people with disabilities, I have engaged in many dialogues with students in which I shared how I dealt with personal challenges as a person with disabilities. For example, we often engage in meaningful and in-depth discussions examining their own perceptions and assumptions about people with disabilities. However, as I have been teaching for many years, I am very conscious about not putting my personal experiences as an individual with disabilities in the foreground of my teaching because I want my students to remember me first as a professor who prepares them to be good teachers with knowledge and skills they will find useful in their own classrooms. From time to time, when I am asked to do guest lectures and other presentations, my personal stories are important tools to convey the main points. However, over the years, I have become more conscious about the extent to which my personal stories become the foreground in these presentations. I always try to embed other research and expert knowledge in them. As an educator, I feel obligated to make my presentations not just motivational speeches but dissemination of knowledge and thought-provoking questions.

Part III Intersection of her story and my story

Reflecting on our experience in academia

As full-time professors, Helen and I have the responsibility of teaching graduate classes, which requires clear verbal communication. My classes are conducted in-person, and this means I need to stand in front of students for about two and a half hours, giving lectures as well as engaging in interactive exchanges with students. All of Helen's classes were converted to online courses before the COVID pandemic, but in the past when her classes were offered in-person, she used her AAC device when she gave class lectures. She talked about the preparation process:

Helen: My course on Computer Application for Special Population used to be an in-person lecture. I would have to prepare a 2-hour and 40-minute lecture, creating scripts and making a PowerPoint on a weekly basis. Several years ago, my classes were changed to an asynchronous online course class. So now students can freely access 1 or 2 weeks of reading materials, post responses on the discussion board, and submit assignments and papers accordingly. Now that the course is asynchronous, I don't have to create as many scripts.

Yoon Joo: It's amazing how you created the verbatim scripts [for each lecture].

Helen: That was the only way I could teach my [in-person] classes.

Yoon Joo: It must have taken a long time for you to prepare your scripts for a 2.5-hour class.

Helen: Absolutely. In the beginning, it would take me the entire week to make the scripts for one class. I would replay each script on the AAC device (Figure 5.1) and keep revising it, so that it sounded natural and made sense. For example, since without commas the AAC device read sentences continuously without pause, I had to add commas where it was appropriate for a pause. I listened to the AAC device several times by myself and rehearsed playing the scripts to make my lectures come out perfectly from the AAC. [laughing]

Although the AAC device has been a very important part of enabling Helen to teach in college classrooms, use of the device has not always been easy, and she has spent many hours creating scripts. Helen also talked about another challenge with the device:

> Due to the nature of the course content, computer application software is constantly being updated or discontinued, and new software and hardware are continuously developed. As a result, it is not possible to use the same scripts from previous semesters. I would have to regularly review and update course contents accordingly.

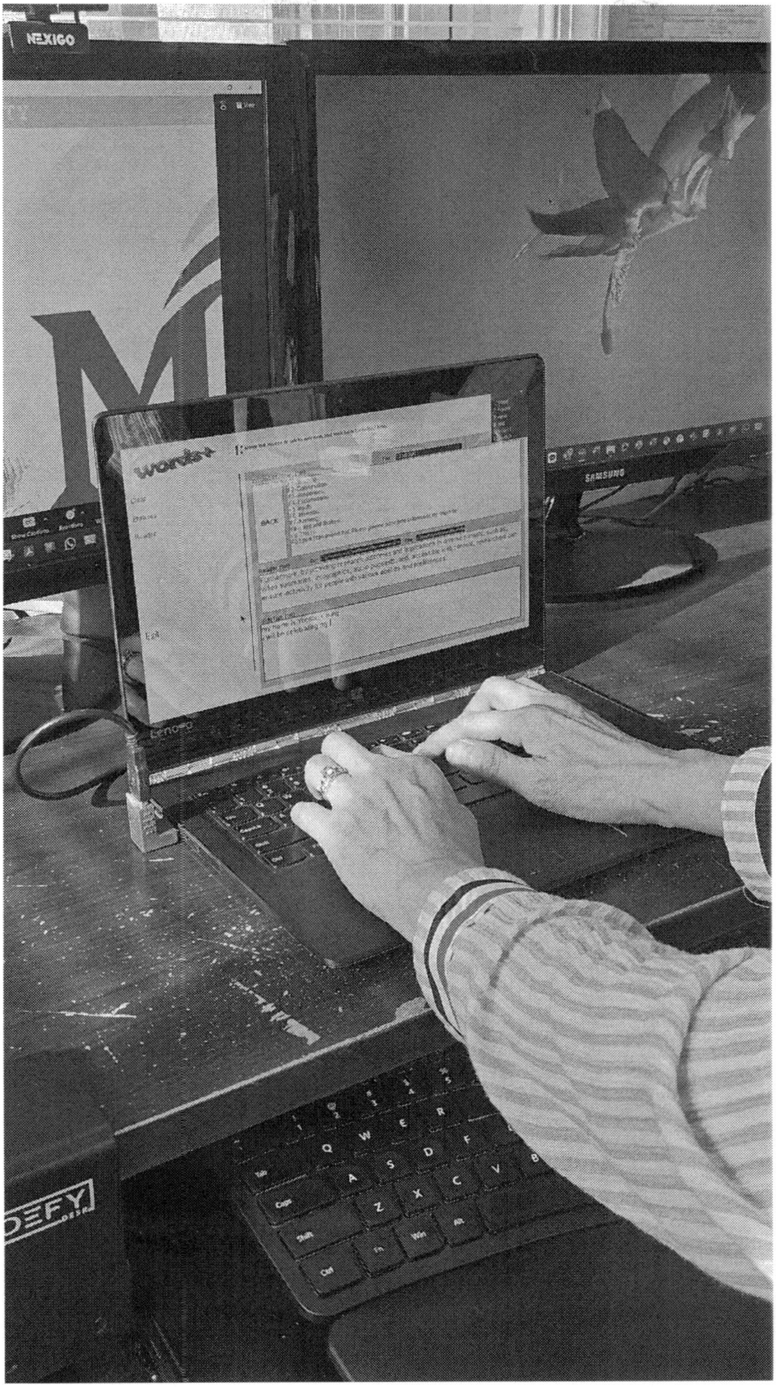

Figure 5.1 Helen utilizing assistive technology to prepare lecture scripts

As I reflected on our conversation about teaching at a university, I realized how Helen and I, as faculty of color with speech impairments, had poured a lot of energy into communicating well, regardless of whether the classes were offered in-person or online. An essential component of teaching is communication, delivering content clearly and effectively. Because of our articulation problems related to cerebral palsy, we had to be more conscious about our ways of speech. At the beginning of my career as a college professor, I always informed students during the first week of classes that it was okay for them to raise their hands and ask me to repeat what I said. I was explicit, explaining to them, apologizing to a certain extent, how likely it was for them not to understand me completely because of my speech impairment and because I am not a native English speaker. Each semester, I was surprised there were only a few instances when the overall flow of the lecture was disrupted because I had to stop and repeat what I had said. Similar to what other colleagues experienced, there were instances in which I had to repeat explanations of difficult concepts, but overall, most students in my classes seemed to understand most of my speech. However, when student evaluations were submitted at the end of the semester, communication was always an area for improvement. During one of the interviews, Helen and I had a conversation about the issue of communication:

Helen: You must have wonderful English pronunciation. My English pronunciation is just not always good.

Yoon Joo: It is difficult to speak English fluently. Perhaps it might be even harder for you since you came to America after graduating high school. I just assume other people understand what I am saying and keep speaking. However, for the first few years, I would always score lower in communication for my annual teaching evaluation by students. The chair would always tell me to improve my communication when we had my annual faculty evaluation.

Helen: I wonder what your chair meant by "improve your communication." Did it mean that you needed to interact more with other professors? Or was the chair literally asking you to improve your speech impairment?

Yoon Joo: That's a great question. I understood it as needing to create my PowerPoint presentations better and improve my teaching skills in terms of explaining things. Perhaps I was just nervous and felt less confident about my teaching during the first few years of teaching in college classrooms.

Helen: Hmm . . . What does it mean for you to improve your PowerPoints? This sounds like vague feedback to me.

Yoon Joo: I didn't realize that before, but you are making a valid point. I've never thought of it in that sense.

During annual conferences with the department chair, who reviewed my performance before I became tenured, communication was always listed as an area for improvement. I just took this feedback for granted without questioning it much. Through my conversation with Helen, I realized I had felt nervous and less confident, powerless to a certain extent, about my teaching during my years as an untenured professor. At the beginning of their careers, many people feel less confident about doing their job. Looking back on that time, my lack of self-confidence might have been connected to how more conscious I was about my disability and language proficiency.

This conversation also made me think about my positionality in relation to power and status. As untenured faculty, I was not in a position of power and was unable to articulate how my communication style was different from others and advocate for myself. I was surprised when I realized that I had stopped giving my speech in the first classes after 20 years of teaching. I am sure my speech impairment has not gotten better over the years. However, as my teaching skills improve and I feel more competent and confident in front of students, I am less self-conscious about my disability.

A unique issue emerged from Helen's story: acknowledging the privileged disability experience

It was incredible how very similar Helen's story was to mine. Both of us went to schools in Korea and came to the United States when we were teenagers. We attended college, earned doctorate degrees in special education, and taught full-time in U.S. colleges. I wonder if we are more accepted, embraced, and given more opportunities to thrive as scholars and professors because our field is special education. As Helen mentioned during the interviews, if we had chosen a field other than special education, we might have encountered more barriers and discrimination. Because we work with students who also have desires to work with individuals with disabilities, the presence of our disabled bodies is more embraced and received in this academic community compared to other fields.

Despite these similarities, our disability experiences have been different. I found it interesting that Helen uses assistive technology to communicate in formal settings because I have not thought about using assistive technology in that aspect. I question whether our work setting has any impact on this matter. I work in a public university setting that often deals with budget challenges. As a faculty member, I rarely receive financial support for tools to incorporate into my teaching, so I am forced to communicate without using any tools. Also, I was really amazed that Helen could drive a car. I learned to drive in high school and obtained a driver's license. However, I got into a car accident the first time I drove on my own. Since then, I have never been brave enough to drive on my own. I realize how different factors affect the extent to which individuals' disabling conditions are manifested.

Helen's story was the most difficult to write out of all the stories in this book. I reflected in-depth on why it was so hard to write her story when we had so many similar experiences. After much reflection, I realized my unsettling and uncomfortable feelings originated from the fact that Helen and I are very privileged compared to many other people with disabilities. Despite having experienced many instances of feeling prejudice and being judged inappropriately by others, our overall lived experiences have been "comfortable" and without major life challenges. We have been pretty successful in our careers. The challenge lay in avoiding the portrayal of a supercrip narrative – a storyline often featuring individuals with disabilities defying the odds and achieving the seemingly impossible. Writing critically about Helen's story was complex because it risked aligning with the supercrip narrative. Through writing Helen's story, I realize how difficult it is to highlight the normalcy of a well-established individual with disabilities without turning their story into propaganda conveying a heartwarming message of "making the impossible possible." When engaging with stories of individuals with disabilities, it becomes crucial to consider a multitude of identifiers, including family dynamics, socioeconomic backgrounds, and the cultural contexts that surround them. This ensures a more nuanced understanding beyond surface-level interpretations of disability experiences.

6 "Life goes on"

The continuous journey of living with a disabled body

This final chapter addresses aspects of lived experiences of disability that are not included in the individual stories. The first section presents what the four women said during the follow-up interviews after having read their own stories. I also reflect upon what it was like to write this book as an autoethnography researcher. Then in the next section, the intersectional experience of other identifiers is described. In addition, the impact of aging is addressed to underscore the dynamic and complex nature of living with physical disabilities. The purpose of this chapter is not to generalize disability experiences but to discuss unique and specific issues that impact the lives of individuals with disabilities.

In our voices: reflecting on our conversations together

Throughout the process of writing this book, I tried to stay true to my commitment to authentically portray the participants' experiences, foregrounding their voices as much as possible. As a part of keeping this commitment, I conducted follow-up interviews with all the participants after I completed writing their chapters. I shared the manuscript of their story with each participant and conducted Zoom interviews after they had reviewed them. Afterward, they shared their reflections. Except for Helen, who is fluent in English, the participants were given Korean translations of their stories.

I asked the women to share what they thought about their stories as well as how it had been for them to participate in the interviews for this book. It was interesting to observe that they commented on different aspects. Helen and Jinju, who had completed their doctorate degrees, made more scholarly comments, likely due to their research experience leading them to read through an academic lens. Helen's comments were more general and touched upon ideological themes such as diversity and inclusion in her reflection:

> I realize once again that people's lives are really special, and individuals' personalities and perspectives are different. I believe that all people work hard and try their best. These days, ideas such as diversity, equity, and inclusion are strongly emphasized. So, I thought about how I need

DOI: 10.4324/9781003609179-6

> to explore these concepts more and appreciate diversity more. While I talked to you, I realized that even more.

Jinju, having just completed her doctoral dissertation at the time of the follow-up interview, felt her chapter reminded her of the books on disability studies that she read during her dissertation research:

> While reading it, I thought it was very well organized. My dissertation was also qualitative research. The way you structured it was very well done through organizing by theme, not simply describing my story in chronological order. The overall structure of my chapter was intriguing to me. Even if you had just arranged my story chronologically like a biography, it would have had its merits. But organizing it by theme, this made it feel like I was reading a disability studies book even though it was my story. Also, our conversations were in Korean, but you wrote my story in English. Then my story in English was translated back into Korean. After several language switches, when I read it, the stories and episodes in the chapter were very familiar to me and stories in my life. But it felt like reading a third-person account. This made me read it more objectively, which felt very refreshing.

Hee-Yeon and Theresa talked more about the way their stories were written, pointing out specific parts they liked. In my conversation with Hee-Yeon, I asked what she thought about how I had conveyed her story:

Hee-Yeon: You did a good job.
Yoon Joo: In what aspect do you think I did well?
Hee-Yeon: I feel like you wrote my story really objectively.
Yoon Joo: As a researcher, I am writing your story, but as an outsider describing your experience, I have been thinking a lot about whether my description is really authentic. That's why I want to hear more about your point of view on your story.
Hee-Yeon: I liked how you wrote about my educational experience in Part 1. Some people might say how amazing it is for me to be successful in this kind of environment [despite many barriers], but I'm glad you just described it as it is without glorifying it as an inspirational story.

Remarkably, Hee-Yeon had noticed that the overall tone I used to describe her experience was not one focused on framing her as a hero, and I was happy to hear this observation. With Theresa, it was interesting how she pinpointed the part I struggled with the most when I was working on her story:

Theresa: You listened to my story and integrated your thoughts into my story. Initially, they [readers] could misinterpret what I said about special education schools. But as I read further along, you truly conveyed my intentions accurately and wrote them accordingly. Overall, I really liked this part.

Yoon Joo: What kind of misunderstanding did you think they might have about when you were talking about special education schools?

Theresa: There was something you wrote about my comments on special education schools being negative. But later, you captured my true intentions, describing my positive memories about activities in special education schools, explaining them well. My intention was to talk about positive experiences in special education schools as well as positive relationships with nondisabled peers in college. I really liked that part.

I had been concerned over what Theresa would say about this section and hoped she would not feel uncomfortable with the way I described her perspective toward special education schools. It took extra effort, trying to convey the message that Theresa's comments were not complaints and criticism, and I was relieved when she said I had presented her thoughts accurately.

Overall, I felt honored and excited to hear from the participants that they enjoyed reading their stories. Most importantly, I was happy to hear they enjoyed the whole interview process and thought my portrait of their lives was authentic and accurate. Hee-Yeon commented:

> I really enjoyed participating in the interviews. Although we aren't strangers, we have not seen each other for a long time and have lived very different lives. So, talking about our lives from childhood to now, I said to myself, "Oh, that's how it was back then." It was very meaningful and rewarding. Through our conversations, I realized that I haven't lived such a bad life after all. And after reading what you wrote about me, it felt like my story clearly illustrated how it is to survive as a disabled woman in Korea. I want to applaud myself for the things I have accomplished.

I was happy to hear that Hee-Yeon felt proud as she read her story. It was validating to learn that the women thought my portrait of their lives showed we were on the same page. Their comments made me realize once again the true value, importance, and power of foregrounding own voices when presenting the lived experiences of disability.

Two sides to autoethnography: connection and discomfort

Profound emotional engagement, including vulnerability and emotional labor, is a critical component of conducting autoethnographic research. Ellis (1999) emphasized the integral role of emotional engagement in autoethnography, highlighting how caring, feeling, passion, and vulnerability are at its center. Autoethnography allows for methodological flexibility, which allowed me, as a researcher, to implement creative approaches in telling the lived experiences of disability and to connect to the participants in a unique way. I was pleasantly surprised by how I was able to build close connections with them given the relatively short period of time I spent with them during my research for this book and even though I had met most of them for the first time during the individual interviews. I had had no prior encounters with the women except for Hee-Yeon, my childhood friend. I am humbled, honored, and grateful that they shared their lives with me, including vulnerable parts that might be uncomfortable to discuss with strangers. After reviewing her chapter, Jinju affirmed the rapport we were able to build through our conversations:

> Reading it after 2 years, I didn't feel like anything was missing. Instead, I thought, "Oh, my, did I really say that back then?" It made me realize, "Wow, I really went into such detail with her," to the point where I thought, "I talked about so many things, even trivial ones."

Her comment indicates that she was very comfortable sharing her life story with me. I certainly experienced a special connection with these women, as we share similar identity markers such as being women with visible disabilities coming from a Korean background. As I wrote each of their stories, I was able to reflect on my own lived experience of disability, and this process of self-reflection has been cathartic and therapeutic, offering me personal growth (Adams et al., 2015).

The most wonderful part of writing this book, as well as a unique aspect of this book, was reflecting and writing on how each of their stories was connected to mine. The participants also appreciated the fact that my personal experience was integrated with their stories. Jinju shared:

> What I liked the most was what I mentioned earlier. The way you matched my story with your thoughts and life experiences. Combining your story as the author with mine made it more persuasive. That's what I liked the most. Personally, after finishing my doctorate degree, I am also considering writing essays about my experiences, so I learned many things [from observing your writing style].

Jinju, who conducted her doctoral study in a field similar to mine, articulated the benefit of autoethnography, describing how this method could empower researchers in highlighting the lived experience of disabilities. Theresa also appreciated the similarity in our thoughts and that this was conveyed in her chapter, saying, "Overall, I felt that what I wanted to convey was quite similar to what you were thinking. Rather than pinpointing specific parts that I liked, I think I liked the entire content as a whole."

As a scholar and individual with disabilities, I utilize autoethnography to explore lived experiences of disability and describe individual stories of past, present, and prospective future experiences of living with disabilities (e.g., Jones, 2020; McKinney, 2018; O'Dea, 2018). There are benefits and privileges to conducting this type of research. At the same time, researchers may experience discomfort and stress as they often share their own deeply personal and potentially painful experiences (Ellis, 2004). This process involves delving into intimate aspects of their lives and can include revisiting traumatic events, personal failures, and private moments. Lourens (2021) argued that narrating difficult portions of life with a disability through the method of autoethnography has the therapeutic power to unlock unconscious experiences, thoughts, and memories. Through writing this book, I have gained a deeper and more nuanced understanding of my own life story (Bantjes & Swartz, 2019). I experienced moments of struggle and discomfort as the participants' stories reminded me of memories I had forgotten. Their memories of stigma and marginalization triggered my own uncomfortable memories that I had not thought about deeply. When Hee-Yeon and Helen shared how they experienced biases and stigma when they first entered mainstream schools, I remembered the stares from peers when I entered middle school. I realized how memory can be active, dynamic, and ever changing.

When individuals with disabilities interact with others who have similar disabilities, they may see their vulnerabilities reflected in them and this may lead to both positive (Silverman et al., 2017) and negative (Ditchman et al., 2013; Paterson et al., 2012) feelings. Conducting this research made me realize how uneasy I can be sometimes when encountering other people with disabilities. I am ashamed of these feelings, but I have come to understand that I am uncomfortable seeing my disabled image reflected back at me. Jinju, whose dissertation involved interviewing other people with disabilities, shared similar feelings, and we talked about this issue:

Jinju: I've heard that people with disabilities may not like meeting other people with disabilities. I first came across this idea while studying disability welfare. When I heard this for the first time, it really struck a chord with me. In classes, I learned that it feels like looking in a mirror, and there's a desire to reject that feeling, which is why there's an underlying psychology of not wanting to face other people with disabilities. Hearing this while I was a university student was particularly beneficial. Because I had always attended only mainstream schools with nondisabled peers, I didn't have many opportunities to become aware of my own [disabled] body. I had only seen people with disabilities in the media, but when I first entered college and met friends with disabilities, including those with severe cerebral palsy, I felt a sense of difference. Seeing those friends, I wondered, "Why do I feel this way?" This uncomfortable feeling bothered me deeply. I thought I was the only one who felt this way. So I couldn't talk to anyone about it, thinking, "I'm a person with a disability; I shouldn't feel this way. Why am I like this? Am I really a bad person?" But hearing that others might have the same feeling,

I realized, "Ah, it's not just me. Other people with disabilities might feel the same way about me." This led me to think that this psychological response might be something that should be acknowledged as normal.

Yoon Joo: As we are talking, I realize that sometimes I also don't particularly feel comfortable associating with other people with disabilities. I am cautious and feel anxious about writing about this uncomfortable feeling. At some points, I have even wondered whether I might be exploiting other people with disabilities for the sake of writing this book. But after discussing it with you, I see you felt the same way and so did I.

Jinju: While conducting interviews for my dissertation, I found that individuals with disabilities who only attended mainstream schools had similar feelings, so I realized I'm not the only one. It wasn't just because you and I attended mainstream schools. Those [participants with disabilities] who attended special education schools also felt similar emotions when they first encountered other peers with disabilities. This shows that it's a common phenomenon. While preparing my dissertation, I realized these feelings are almost universal. Therefore, it might be necessary for someone to publicize it more, so that people are aware of it.

As I wrote these women's stories, I felt uneasy when their perspectives on their lived experience of disability differed from mine. I was uncomfortable when they described their disabilities in a positive light, not talking too much about challenges, since it seemed their reflections lacked critical reflection. However, if they focused too much on negative aspects, sharing gloomy or pessimistic views on disability, I also felt uneasy. Since being reflexive and critically examining one's own position, biases, and influence on the research can be complex and demanding (Finlay, 2002), I wonder if this uncomfortable feeling is an unavoidable and challenging part of conducting autoethnographic research. To some extent, I wonder if other identifiers, such as SES, influenced the participants' perceptions of their disabilities. While reflecting on the interview process, my own privileged socioeconomic background led me to have feelings of guilt and discomfort. It took some time for me to come to terms with this feeling of guilt I had as a researcher and writer of this book and to acknowledge the intersectionality of my identity.

Intersection of multiple identities in disability experiences

Living as women with disabilities

Each person has multiple identities, and each identity can be associated with experiences of privilege or oppression. Kimberlé Crenshaw (1991), a key figure in the development of the concept of intersectionality, emphasized how race, gender, class, and other social identities intersect to create unique experiences of oppression and discrimination for women of color. When considering the lives of individuals with disabilities, it is very likely for disability identity to "cancel out" other qualities and reduce the complex identity of a disabled person to one attribute (Garland-Thomson, 1997). Therefore, the framework of intersectionality is important in illuminating the complex and interwoven ways in which individuals with disabilities experience discrimination and marginalization. Some may face multiple, interacting forms of inequity. The stories of the women in this book certainly illustrate how their experiences of disability have been influenced by the intersectionality of multiple identifiers.

Women with disabilities often face multiple layers of stigma and discrimination since the intersection of gender and disability results in compounded disadvantages. During the interviews, Hee-Yeon clearly articulated how the intersection of her identifiers, gender and disability, affected her educational experience:

> First of all, for disabled women in Korea, social expectations for their lives are not that high. So parents were more likely to believe that even if girls with disabilities learned something in school, it wouldn't help, and their educational advancement was considered useless. That's why my mom didn't really intend to educate me much.
>
> In my opinion, since our family didn't have enough money, I wondered whether my mom wasn't very interested in pushing me to go to more prestigious schools because she wasn't sure if it was worth it to invest resources. My mom wasn't very interested in my studies. So, looking back, I think I just continued in my studies without support from my school even though my school couldn't provide much support. There were quite a few cases like that.
>
> If I had been a boy, the situation might have been a bit different. Typically, girls with disabilities don't get as much attention. In the case of a boy I knew who had a similar physical condition to mine, his whole family helped him a lot with his school life even though he wasn't very good at studying. Of course, things have changed a lot now, but still, I sometimes think that if I weren't a girl but a boy, I might be able to earn a bit more than I do now.

Hee-Yeon's experience as a girl with disabilities may no longer accurately represent the current era's expectations since Korean society has become less patriarchal. Korea was historically considered a patriarchal society that favored sons over daughters because they were seen as carriers of the family lineage and were expected to provide financial support for their aging parents. However, recent studies indicate a significant shift in these traditional preferences (Choi & Hwang, 2020; Chung & Das Gupta, 2007). Increasingly, parents in South Korea prefer daughters over sons due to evolving societal values and economic considerations. This shift is reflected in the declining sex ratio at birth and more families expressing a preference for daughters (Korea Joongang Daily, 2023). Still, Hee-Yeon's story highlights how the intersection of disability and gender can manifest depending on the sociocultural context of a certain historical time. If she had been born in the more modern era, in which Korean society is less patriarchal, she might not have felt such a significant degree of marginalization.

When describing the experiences of disabled women, it is necessary to address topics such as singleness, dating, and marriage, as these areas significantly impact the personal and social experiences of individuals. The intersectionality of disability and gender affects personal relationships, social expectations, and societal norms. The marital status of the four women in this book is diverse, ranging from being married for almost 30 years to being in a long-term relationship to being single with past dating experience. Their lives represent a wide range of stories, similar to those of the typical population of nondisabled women, and their views on dating and marriage are not very different either. However, their disability identity may have significant impacts on their romantic relationships.

Individuals with disabilities are construed as nonsexual and undeserving or incapable of having satisfying sexual relationships (Rainey, 2011). Contrary to the conventional wisdom and low societal expectations for women with physical disabilities in Korea, Helen is one woman who has completely taken on the maternal responsibilities in her family (Lee & Oh, 2005). However, she shared an anecdote about a member of her husband's family who had made a negative assumption about her when her husband first introduced her to his family and expressed his decision to marry her:

> My husband has many siblings. He has three older sisters and a younger brother. My husband is the fourth child. Many years later, I heard that the husband of his second oldest sister thought. . . since I was studying abroad at that time, he assumed that only financially well-off people could study abroad. He suspected that my husband wanted to marry me for my financial status.

This initial reaction illustrates the biased assumption that women with disabilities are less able-bodied and less valuable in the context of dating and finding a mate (Milligan & Neufeldt, 2001). Seemingly at odds with this kind of assumption, Helen's parents were also initially against the marriage. They objected to the 6-year age difference between Helen and her husband; she was 24 years old, and he was already in his 30s. She said, "My parents thought they had sent their innocent girl to America to study, and a man in his 30s was trying to take advantage of her." One might assume that when a man wants to marry a woman with disabilities, only his side of the family would oppose the marriage. But in Helen's case, the opposition came from both the bride's and groom's sides. Her story illustrates how women with disabilities can be viewed in prejudiced ways even when going through the typical process of two individuals being united.

In contrast to Helen and Theresa, Jinju and Hee-Yeon are single in their 40s after having very few dating experiences. They talked about the challenges of dating and finding a life partner. Jinju explained her decision to not think about dating and marriage:

> Although I have good memories from that time [first romantic relationship in 20s], the relationship with my ex-boyfriend ended badly and became a bit of a wound for me. As a result, that experience made me more resolute. The desire not to get hurt again has strengthened my emotional walls over the years, especially from my 30s into my 40s. It's often said that as nondisabled people get older, it becomes harder for them to date and marry due to overthinking and increased worries. For me, this is compounded by my own experiences and the situation of my disability, which seem to intensify my defensive mechanisms as I age.
>
> Moreover, I wasn't naturally inclined toward romantic relationships to begin with, and my last experience was in my 20s. So having been single for over 15 years, any small inclination I had toward romance seems to have diminished even further. There aren't many single men around me who could be potential partners. Even if there are, it's hard to tell if they are genuinely interested in me or if I'm just imagining things. I worry about getting excited for no reason and making a move, only to realize it was a mistake.

When I heard this, I felt heavyhearted thinking that my pessimistic perspective on dating, which I wrote about in her story, might have further convinced her not to pursue dating. Even though there may be barriers and stigma associated with physical disabilities, I didn't want her to stay discouraged and stop dating:

Jinju: I really liked the part about dating and the marriage stories you wrote in my chapter because it didn't just end with my story. You also wrote about the parts we both empathized with. Once again, I felt, "Oh, I could see it that way." What I also empathized with was the part where you mentioned you also totally avoid dating and such. I think that's how I am now.

Yoon Joo: Oh, I was like that in my 20s, but I started dating after I turned 40.

Jinju: Oh, really?

Yoon Joo: I started dating late. Dating at an older age made me realize that with so many important things in life, getting hurt by a man isn't a big deal.

Jinju: I guess you could really think that way.

Yoon Joo: In my 20s, I was afraid of facing the reality of dating associated with stereotypes and negative assumptions about disabilities. But when I reached my 40s, I realized that with so many difficult things in life, if you break up with a boyfriend, it's no big deal anymore.

Jinju: That's true.

Yoon Joo: So, don't build too many walls and avoid dating experiences. . . . Hearing that you blocked thoughts about dating makes me feel really sad.

I completely understand Jinju's decision and realize there are similar yet different ways our intersectional identities of disability and gender affect dating and marriage.

Hee-Yeon, who had experience dating both men with disabilities and nondisabled men, said the experiences were not particularly enjoyable:

> First of all, my disabled boyfriends thought of me as someone who they could brag about. They wanted to show off that they had a "great catch" [successful and less disabled] like me. They thought that since they had disabilities, they should date someone they considered inferior to them, but meeting someone like me made them feel superior. And with nondisabled men, it feels like they aren't dating me because they genuinely like me. After some time, it started to feel less like I was their girlfriend but more like they were doing volunteer work. At first, they treated me very well, but it felt strange to me somehow. And unless it was unavoidable, they tried to keep my presence as their girlfriend a secret from their friends. Maybe it's just because I dated only those kinds of guys, but I could never make it past a year in a relationship, so I thought maybe I can't have a relationship.

Our conversation about romantic relationships moved further to the following:

Hee-Yeon: Since I was young, my parents have always told me to live alone and not even think about getting married. I think that made me instinctively push people away.

Yoon Joo: I'm the same. My parents also told me to live alone and not date, so I didn't have my first relationship until I was over 40. I think I started too late. It might have been easier to date if I had started dating at a younger age.

Through this conversation, I realized how parents' expectations can implicitly and explicitly affect our views toward dating and marriage. While listening to Hee-Yeon and Jinju, I, now single in my 50s, wholeheartedly empathized with them. It occurred to me that the societal messages we received unconsciously and the messages from our parents, as well as social expectations, have shaped our perspectives on dating and marriage. Women with visible disabilities may be judged as flawed or defective as romantic partners because they do not conform to the narrow socially accepted descriptions of physical attractiveness (Gill, 1996; Milligan & Neufeldt, 2001). These physical differences may be understood as constituting "visible difference" and have been defined by Kent and Thompson (2002) as "potentially noticeable differences in appearance that are not culturally sanctioned" (p. 103). Carol Gill, a polio survivor, researcher, and self-described cultural revolutionist, articulated two factors – aesthetics and function – to explain the romantic disadvantages of women with disabilities (Gill, 1996). Milligan and Neufeldt (2001) argued that actual and/or perceived rejection may lead some people with disabilities to retreat from intimacy, ergo, the adoption of a nonsexual lifestyle.

Theresa's experience and perspective are different from those of the three other women, and her story reflects the current trend among many young Koreans. Theresa has been dating her boyfriend for about nine years, and there is no concrete plan to get married in the near future:

> In the past, I used to think that I needed to get married quickly, probably up until my 20s. I guess the reason I thought that way was I had a strong desire to become independent. Back then, I just thought, "Oh, if I get married, I can live on my own quickly." But now, as I'm starting different projects and progressing in my work, I wonder if marriage is really necessary. After all, marriage would bring certain restrictions compared to now. So I'm questioning whether I really need to get married. As for dating, I'm currently still in a relationship.

Many young Koreans are increasingly choosing not to get married due to several factors such as economic challenges and the growing appeal of single life (McDonald, 2023). Theresa's viewpoint reflects the current perspectives of young Koreans who no longer see marriage as a necessity but view it as potentially restrictive. The diverse perspectives and experiences in the context of dating and marriage among the women in this book illustrate no singular pattern. Their stories are varied and deeply personal. There is no uniform perspective. Similar to nondisabled women, our decisions about being single or married are influenced not just by our disabilities but also by age, social expectations, cultural norms, and individual circumstances.

The uncomfortable truth about the intersection of disability and socioeconomic background

Among the diverse intersections of identifiers in individuals, socioeconomic background may have the most significant impact on lived experiences of disability. Access to economic resources and the subsequent opportunities shape social class habitus, which, in turn, interacts with disability to influence individuals' sense of purpose, including their thoughts, choices, and feelings about careers and life goals (Vaccaro et al., 2019). If individuals with disabilities come from a low socioeconomic background, their life experience is first changed by the fact they have scarce resources and less access to different opportunities. As I wrote about the women's stories, the most striking aspect was the significant impact of SES on their lives, and this issue was almost universal across the book.

In the stories of Theresa and Hee-Yeon, the economic resources of their families seemed to influence the range of opportunities they had. Living in a rural area, Theresa experienced limited access to and opportunity for inclusive education and special education services that were appropriately suited to her needs. Even though she did not reveal the details of the socioeconomic background of her family, several of the stories she shared implied her family did not have enough resources to live in more urban areas (which have higher living costs) where Theresa could have had more opportunities for inclusive education. Hee-Yeon had a strong desire to study abroad and was academically capable and motivated to advance her education, but she faced financial barriers that prevented her from studying abroad. Her family did not have the financial means to support her in pursuing an advanced degree. She had no choice but to stay in Korea. As adults, both Theresa and Hee-Yeon are capable of driving and Theresa has passed her driving test, but owning a car is a luxury for them. Also, Hee-Yeon is clearly able to live alone, outside of her parents' house, as a typical adult; however, it is financially challenging to afford a place of her own because housing prices in Seoul are very high.

On the other hand, Helen's and Jinju's parents were able to financially support them, which opened up more opportunities. While Jinju didn't go abroad for an advanced degree, she participated in a few short-term study abroad programs. Her parents could financially afford to establish a scholarship at the university she attended for the purpose of supporting a college student who could be Jinju's roommate and help her with living in the dorm. Helen's parents were able to send her to a university in the United States. Helen continued to graduate school and completed a doctorate degree with financial support from her parents. Helen clearly articulated her privilege:

> The support from my parents was significant in allowing me to grow up without difficulties, in Korea as well as in the U.S. Their financial support made it possible for me to study even after coming here [United States]. I believe that our lives do not completely represent the experiences of people with disabilities in Korea. As Koreans with disabilities, our lives are greatly influenced by favorable environmental factors, for which we are very grateful. Therefore, my story cannot fully represent the experiences of people with disabilities in Korea.

Helen's story illustrates how people with disabilities do not always feel oppressed and powerless. Because of other identifiers such as SES and access to education and employment, individuals can be in a position of privilege. I have to admit that SES encompasses resources for further educational opportunities and financial security as well as privileges and quality of life attributes. Even though all of the women and I had similar capacities to succeed, as a person in a privileged position, I felt uncomfortable facing the inconvenient truth that our lived experiences had evolved differently because of our families' socioeconomic backgrounds. This sense of discomfort led me to question my eligibility to write this book and made me cautious about writing on this issue. Despite this sense of inadequacy and uneasiness, I recognize how important it is to speak honestly about my position of privilege and to acknowledge these differences in order to understand the full spectrum of disability experience. It is my hope that acknowledging the intersection of disability and SES can help create more meaningful stories with nuance and complexity.

One critical takeaway from reflecting on the intersection of disability and SES is the clear reminder of the danger of overlooking the socioeconomic background of individuals with disabilities when addressing their success in mainstream society. Without considering SES, there is a tendency to overemphasize the hard work of disabled individuals in becoming well-adjusted and successful, while failing to recognize how systemic oppression influences their access to resources, navigation of inequitable social systems, and self-understanding within the context of dominant norms and values (Hill-Collins & Bilge, 2016). Neglecting the role of SES can lead to an incomplete understanding of the barriers faced by individuals with disabilities and the support they need to succeed. Intersectionality shows that the discrimination faced by individuals with disabilities can be amplified by other aspects of their identity.

Normalizing disability experience while highlighting unique aspects

Typical and atypical aspects of aging with disabilities

Aging is a universal phenomenon that affects every individual. Many people expect the aging process to begin later in life and are taken aback when it starts earlier than anticipated. In particular, individuals with physical disabilities are more likely to experience accelerated aging compared to their nondisabled counterparts. People with disabilities have various problems associated with premature aging as their biological age is higher than their chronological age (Molton & Yorkston, 2017). Age-related physiological changes occur earlier in adults with cerebral palsy, and these individuals experience a higher prevalence of secondary conditions such as pain, osteoporosis, and musculoskeletal and joint problems, compared to age-matched adults without cerebral palsy (Mudge et al., 2016). The lived experiences of people who have grown older with their disability are significantly different from the experiences of people who become disabled at an older age (CPA,

2016). Even though aging with disabilities occurs in a unique context, what happens to these individuals with aging is not yet well understood (Westwood & Carey, 2018).

As I listened to the women's stories, and as I am going through my own aging process, I felt it was essential to include a discussion of aging in this book about the lived experiences of disability. Personally, aging with disabilities has become a very important issue in my life. For most of my life, I considered myself pretty healthy – I had no allergies or major health issues. My best friend used to tease me by saying I was healthier in my disabled body than she was in her able body. Because of cerebral palsy, I walk slower than others and my gait is different, but I felt confident in maneuvering the world around me until my late 30s. I was caught by surprise when I began to feel pain in my right knee at the age of 38 while walking and climbing stairs. When the pain first started, I had planned to see a regular orthopedist in my neighborhood, but my friend pointed out that it might be more appropriate for me to see a physical medicine and rehabilitation doctor. Until my friend shared this insight, I hadn't considered that my disability might be connected, but looking back, I realized I had been thinking of my disability as separate from my overall health condition.

With my friend's help, I found a pediatric orthopedic surgeon who specializes in cerebral palsy. After taking X-rays, the doctor informed me the pain was associated with signs of arthritis in my knee and prescribed an ankle foot orthosis. Even when I was young, I had never worn any orthoses so this experience made me think about my disability in a whole new way. After several months, when the ankle foot orthosis did not completely resolve the knee pain, I was referred to another orthopedist who discovered my cartilage was worn away. I underwent arthroscopic surgery and the pain disappeared. Although the surgery alleviated the knee pain, as I age, I have started to feel pain in other places such as my back and wrists. More than anything, when walking outside or using public transportation, I find myself being more cautious with my steps and worrying more about falling compared to when I was younger.

The women shared their experiences of age-related changes and health issues due to their physical disabilities. For example, there is a relatively high prevalence of symptomatic cervical spinal stenosis among adults with primarily spastic cerebral palsy who complain of new-onset pain or changes in motor function (Hung et al., 2020). At the time of the follow-up interview, Theresa was in the middle of recovery and rehabilitation after surgery involving screws in her neck due to nerve damage and cervical stenosis. She was in good spirits and working continuously on her recovery. When I asked her what aging means to her, this was her response:

Theresa: The idea that the body ages? I've already been living with the thought that my body isn't typical for my age since my 20s.

Yoon Joo: In what way?

Theresa: I started having spinal issues back then, and gradually, my ability to walk has deteriorated. But at that time, I ignored it and overworked my body, and now, I feel like my body is in worse condition than it was back then.

Yoon Joo: I see. Everyone I've interviewed, including myself, has lived life so intensely that the aging process seems to have come faster than expected.

Theresa: Yes, so now I'm a bit scared. I don't think being in your 40s is that old, but my physical age seems to be showing much more than that. While living as a member of this society, it feels like my ability to function is gradually shrinking – at an age when it shouldn't be. I can't help but think that way sometimes.

Theresa articulated clearly the harsh reality of aging with disability. Even though the physical effects of aging were not as significant for them as for Theresa, Helen and Hee-Yeon were also dealing with challenges associated with their aging bodies. In her late 40s, when Helen was experiencing severe shoulder pain, her doctor prescribed Botox treatment for relief. Since then, Botox treatment has become important to Helen for pain management and reducing muscle spasticity. She described the physical challenges she has faced as she gets older and the benefits of receiving Botox treatment:

Helen: Physically, I definitely feel it's getting harder. Especially for people with CP, it seems like physical aging happens faster. Things like shoulder pain, neck pain, stiffness in the body. . . . CP people use their muscles a lot, so . . .

Yoon Joo: It feels like we're aging too quickly. Do you still get Botox these days?

Helen: Yes, I make sure to get it once a month. I don't think I could live without it now.

Yoon Joo: How does Botox help you?

Helen: First, it reduces muscle pain. Since Botox relaxes the muscles, it decreases muscle pain and also stops the face from grimacing, which greatly improves my quality of life.

Yoon Joo: How long have you been getting Botox?

Helen: About 7 to 8 years, maybe 8 years. I started getting it for my face about 3 to 4 years ago, but initially, I was only getting it in my shoulders and other areas.

Yoon Joo: Did you start getting it because your shoulders were hurting?

Helen: Yes, the muscle pain was so severe that I was looking for a solution, and I found out that Botox treatment helps with muscle relaxation.

Helen also shared that she feels more comfortable articulating her speech as the Botox helps her muscles relax. Similar to Helen, Hee-Yeon has also dealt with physical challenges such as back and wrist pain. She commented how her walking had become less stable and she was falling down more frequently compared to when she was in her 20s. When she was younger, she could climb the stairs in subway stations without holding on to the railing, but in the past few years, she has needed to hang on to the railing when climbing the stairs. The spasticity in her neck due to cerebral palsy has led to discomfort and pain in her neck and shoulder as she becomes older. She has visited many doctors, but most treatments, such as Botox, are not covered by health insurance. Hee-Yeon has begun to face the important dilemma of how much to spend on taking care of her aging disabled body given the mediocre income she earns as an editor in a publishing company, not a very high-paying job in Korea. She said, "I feel pain everywhere, even in my ears. And my medical expenses are incredibly high now, so I'm constantly thinking about how to earn enough to cover them. Lately, as I get older, I've been really curious about how other people are managing and living their lives."

Aging for these women not only involves physical aspects of their own disabled bodies but also affects the dynamics of their relationships with others, including parents. Jinju, who is the most physically disabled of the women in this book, reflected on the changing dynamics of her relationship with her mom as they both age:

> Because I have a disability, my physical condition [in my 40s] is almost similar to my parents', unlike nondisabled people at my age. I often say things like "Ouch, my joints hurt" when I am with my mom. Sitting in a wheelchair for long periods causes pain in my hips and pelvis. At the end of the day, we're both completely exhausted. My mom is always talking about her knee pain or how something else hurts. She jokingly tells me, "A young person [referring to herself in a sarcastic way] in her seventies is showing off wrinkles to someone in her forties". When she says things like that, I start thinking that aging will only get harder. I often reflect on how my physical condition is becoming more like my mom's as I get older.
>
> Despite my mom always thinking she has to take care of me, she's now over 70, has presbyopia, and needs glasses because she can't see small things well anymore. Her senses are dulling, and it's psychologically very hard for her. I've experienced many physical limitations for a long time due to my disability. I faced these challenges early on, so I tell my mom, "Mom, you need to accept it just like people with disabilities accept their limitations. You're not alone in this. Everyone experiences these things as they age. It's the same for everyone. Mom, your daughter struggles with dropping things all the time. Remember how you encouraged me to overcome it? Now you need to do the same." Then she says, "You're still young, you don't know what it's like to be old," and gives me a playful bop on the head. We often have these kinds of conversations.

Since Jinju's physical disability is significant and requires a lot of physical assistance, she has become concerned about her aging mother. Her mother takes care of many aspects of her daily activities during periods when she cannot find disability support workers. Jinju shared that it has always been challenging to find new support workers, and as her mother is in her 70s, it has also become more challenging for her to take care of Jinju, so the aging process has affected both Jinju and her mother.

Hee-Yeon is able to live completely independently, not needing much physical support to carry out daily activities though there are some physical challenges associated with aging. However, as she becomes older, she has noticed that her articulation issue related to cerebral palsy is worsening, and it is harder for people to understand her speech, including her mother. As her mother's hearing becomes worse as she gets older, their verbal communication has become more challenging:

> Lately, what I worry about the most is that, while I can manage other things at home, my speech impairment isn't getting any better. Nowadays, my mom often can't understand what I'm saying as her hearing deteriorates, even though my dad is fine. Communication is really important in social relationships, you know. I still believe that face-to-face conversations are the most important. But as my speech impairment worsens, I feel like my social relationships are gradually diminishing. Meeting new people has become really daunting. . . . I can see that they have trouble understanding me, and it makes it hard for me to speak up.

Hee-Yeon shared that communication had become a pressing issue especially because she often needs to meet with new people in her freelance editing jobs. Such unique aspects of aging with disabilities emerged across the four women's stories.

As illustrated in these stories of lived experiences, aging for individuals with physical disabilities includes both the normal aspects of aging and other unique issues associated with disabilities. Figuring out ways of successful aging for adults with disabilities is beyond the scope of this book, as the four individuals and I are just in the middle of the aging process and do not know yet how to age well in our disabled bodies. Facing the reality of an aging body has come sooner than expected, bringing newness, challenges, and concerns. However, we manage not to avoid disability and are directly confronting this new reality, contemplating how to live well with our changing bodies, and finding new solutions. For instance, Helen's approach has included taking tai chi lessons and working out with a personal trainer once a week after realizing the importance of exercise to her pain management. Additionally, observing our aging parents, we are thinking about how we can live independently without relying on them. The journey of living with a disability is not static; it is dynamic, evolving, and constantly changing.

Striving to live with aspirations but refusing to be inspirations

Traditionally disability has been viewed as either a highly positive or highly negative phenomenon. Disability is described as the object of pity or charity, and disabled individuals are represented as sad and helpless, needing assistance from well-meaning nondisabled people. At the other end of the spectrum, discourses on disability are focused on overcoming impairment through hard work, and these type of stories are "supercrip" narratives (Clare, 2009; Young, 2014). In supercrip narratives, disabled people who are simply living their lives become symbols of inspiration (Clare, 2009) and are presented as extraordinary for doing something ordinary that nondisabled people would not celebrate as an achievement. It is easier and more comfortable to focus on supercrip narratives since inspirational narratives, cheerfulness, and sameness are favored in this world (Watermeyer, 2017). Riley (2005) asserted that the "sadcrip" and the supercrip are two sides of the same coin since they are part of a single discourse identifying impairment as tragedy. Representation of disability as either one or the other is based on the belief that achievement contradicts disability (Clare, 2009).

According to Kama (2004), there are two types of supercrip narratives. The regular supercrip narrative focuses on individuals with disabilities who are praised for doing something ordinary based on the ableist assumption that they cannot do things like everyone else. The second type is the glorified supercrip narrative. This is a representation of people with disabilities who "achieve feats that even non-disabled persons rarely attempt" (Kama, 2004, p. 454). Examples may include those who participate in the Paralympics or become world-renowned musicians. Wendell (1996) argued that focus on the achievements of disabled individuals from privileged race, gender, and socioeconomic backgrounds is likely to create "otherness" for the majority of people with disabilities. Supercrip narratives are problematic because these representations center around a disabled individual's attitude, hard work, and perseverance instead of challenging social barriers and systematic oppression in an ableist society (Schalk, 2016).

Stepping away from supercrip narratives, the main focus of this book is to normalize the experiences of individuals with disabilities while yet highlighting unique aspects of living with disability. Many people with disabilities live ordinary lives day in and day out. I embarked on this project with the purpose of describing the ordinary lives of women with physical disabilities like myself. While many may find our stories inspirational, our stories are about typical experiences. Theresa's comment illustrates how lived experiences of disability can be ordinary:

> [When I read my chapter], it didn't quite feel like my own story. Although it is my life and it's definitely what I've lived through, seeing it written by someone else made me think that there must be other people living similar lives. It made me feel like it's not just my story alone.

When I shared with her the initial draft of her story, Hee-Yeon also noticed that it was not written as an inspirational story and understood my intention of not making this book a supercrip narrative. I was excited to receive this feedback because it validated my efforts to be on the same page, trying to not focus on the successes of disabled individuals but describing their experiences authentically and meaningfully.

I acknowledge the four women featured in this book have made remarkable accomplishments despite barriers and challenges. They are fighters and advocates, paving the way while dealing with bias and prejudice due to their visible disabilities. I feel honored and privileged to share their stories celebrating their resilience, aspirations, and strength. This book is intended not to describe them as symbols of inspiration, but as individuals striving to live their lives authentically and meaningfully with all their best efforts. Cameron (2024) suggested that representation of disability be grounded in disabled people's individual and collective voices to make sense of the disability experience. The focus on individuality is also important in creating narratives about people with disabilities (Schalk, 2016). Lived experiences of disability need to be described in a more holistic and diverse manner, as disability is an integrated aspect of an individual's identity (Harvey, 2015). It is more appropriate to view the presence of disability in a person's life as shaping all aspects of the person rather than as something to pity or overcome the traditional societal response.

Throughout the writing process, I grappled with how to celebrate these women's accomplishments without falling into the trap of creating supercrip narratives. Since I incorporated the autoethnographic approach, I also integrated my life stories throughout the book. Therefore, my biggest challenge was balancing both the ordinary and extraordinary moments in our lives. These four women and I share common experiences related to having visible disabilities, but our stories highlight the varied experiences of women with disabilities and feature the multiple layers of complexity and subtle nuances related to multiple identifiers, such as gender, SES, and cultural context. Our journeys of living with disability are unique, dynamic, and evolving. As the four women with disabilities shared their stories, I observed how they were all trying to live their lives with aspiration, striving to achieve personal goals and ambitions, while rejecting the role of inspiration for others. They continue to set up new goals in their lives and continue to work toward achieving their goals. For example, Hee-Yeon continues to study the Japanese language and culture to become an expert in editing Japanese literature. As she recovers from major surgery, Theresa has signed up to take surfing classes specifically designed for individuals with disabilities. Also, her next plan is to pursue a doctorate in disability studies.

To be aspirational but refuse to be inspirational is about recognizing and valuing the true capability, potential, and resilience of individuals with disabilities. It emphasizes the need to shift from viewing disability through a lens of pity or undue admiration to one of respect and genuine acknowledgment of personal and professional achievement. Disabled people deserve to be seen in an integrated, holistic way and to be recognized as having as much diversity as characterizes the human condition (Harvey, 2015). Our stories are not just about disability but about life and the multitude ways in which we navigate it with support from family members, friends, and community. The stories in this book are written to encourage other disabled individuals to embrace their right to be themselves, live authentically, and assert their right to be seen and heard despite the barriers and stigma associated with disabilities. As this book comes to an end, it is important to remember once again how the journey of living with disabilities is diverse and complex, shaped by multiple and intersecting identities. This book celebrates the individuality of these women, highlighting the fact that their lives are not defined solely by their disabilities. Understanding disability requires a multifaceted approach that recognizes the unique challenges and triumphs faced by individuals. By embracing the full spectrum of these lived experiences, disability can be viewed not as a limitation but as one of the many aspects that contribute to the rich diversity of human life.

References

Adams, T. E., Jones, S. H., & Ellis, C. (2015). *Autoethnography: Understanding qualitative research*. Oxford University Press.

Bantjes, J., Swartz, L., & Botha, J. (2019). Troubling stereotypes: South African elite disability athletes and the paradox of (self-)representation. *Journal of Community Psychology*, *47*(4), 819–832. https://doi.org/10.1002/jcop.22155

Cameron, C. (2024). Some things never seem to change: Further towards an affirmation model. *Disability & Society*, *39*(7), 1890–1895. https://doi.org/10.1080/09687599.2023.2295799

Centre for Policy on Ageing. (2016). *Rapid review: Diversity in older age – disability*. https://www.ageuk.org.uk/globalassets/age-uk/documents/reports-and-publications/reports-and-briefings/equality-and-human-rights/rb_may16_cpa_rapid_review_diversity_in-_older_age_disability.pdf

Choi, E. J., & Hwang, J. (2020). Transition of son preference: Evidence from South Korea. *Demography*, *57*(2), 627–652. https://doi.org/10.1007/s13524-020-00863-x

Chung, W., & Das Gupta, M. (2007). The decline of son preference in South Korea: The roles of development and public policy. *Population and Development Review*, *33*(4), 757–783. https://doi.org/10.1111/j.1728-4457.2007.00196.x

Clare, E. (2009). *Exile and pride: Disability, queerness, and liberation*. Cambridge, MA: South End Press.

Crenshaw, K. (1991). Mapping the margins: Intersectionality, identity politics, and violence against women of color. *Stanford Law Review*, *43*(6), 1241–1299. https://doi.org/10.2307/1229039

Ditchman, N., Werner, S., Kosyluk, K., Jones, N., Elg, B., & Corrigan, P. W. (2013). Stigma and intellectual disability: Potential application of mental illness research. *Rehabilitation Psychology*, *58*(2), 206–216. https://doi.org/10.1037/a0032466

Ellis, C. (1999). Heartful autoethnography. *Qualitative Health Research*, *9*(5), 669–683. https://doi.org/10.1177/104973299129122153

Ellis, C. (2004). *The ethnographic I: A methodological novel about autoethnography*. Walnut Creek, CA: AltaMira Press.

Finlay, L. (2002). "Outing" the researcher: The provenance, process and practice of reflexivity. *Qualitative Health Research*, *12*(4), 531–545. https://doi.org/10.1177/104973202129120052

Garland-Thomson, R. (1997). *Extraordinary bodies: Figuring physical disability in American culture and literature*. Columbia University Press.

Gill, C. J. (1996). Dating and relationship issues . . . some of the difficulties encountered by women with disabilities. *Sexuality & Disability*, *14*(3), 183–190. https://doi.org/10.1007/bf02590076

Harvey, C. (2015). What's disability got to do with it? Changing constructions of Oscar Pistorius before and after the death of Reeva Steenkamp. *Disability & Society*, *30*(2), 299–304. https://doi.org/10.1080/09687599.2014.1000511

Hill-Collins, P., & Bilge, S. (2016). *Intersectionality*. Cambridge: Polity Press.

Hung, C. W., Matsumoto, H., Ball, J. R., Plachta, S., Dutkowsky, J. P., Kim, H., Hyman, J. E., Riew, K. D., & Roye, D. P. (2020). Symptomatic cervical spinal stenosis in spastic cerebral palsy. *Developmental Medicine & Child Neurology*, *62*, 1147–1153. https://doi.org/10.1111/dmcn.14607

Jones, P. (2020). On being a zebra: Negotiating a professional identity whilst coping with a rare and recurrent illness. *The Qualitative Report*, *25*(6), 1713–1720. https://doi.org/10.46743/2160-3715/2020.4295

Kama, A. (2004). Supercrips versus the pitiful handicapped: Reception of disabling images by disabled audience members. *Communications*, *29*(4), 447–466.

Kent, G., & Thompson, A. (2002). The development and maintenance of shame in disfigurement: Implications for treatment. In P. Gilbert & J. Miles (Eds.), *Body shame: Conceptualisation, research and treatment* (pp. 103–116). Hove: Brunner Routledge.

Korea Joongang Daily. (2023, March 3). Koreans now prefer daughters over sons as society changes. *Korea JoongAng Daily*. https://koreajoongangdaily.joins.com/2023/03/03/national/socialAffairs/korea-daughter-son/20230303164033873.html?detailWord=

Lee, E. O., & Oh, H. (2005). A wise wife and good mother: Reproductive health and maternity among women with disability in South Korea. *Sexuality and Disability*, *23*, 121–144. https://doi.org/10.1007/s11195-005-6728-y

Lourens, H. (2021). Supercripping the academy: The difference narrative of a disabled academic. *Disability & Society*, *36*(8), 1205–1220. https://doi.org/10.1080/09687599.2020.1794798

McDonald, A. (2023, November 4). 4 reasons Korea's younger generation refuses to get married. *Koreaboo*. https://www.koreaboo.com/lists/korea-young-generation-refuses-get-married-reaons-yonhap-news/

McKinney, E. M. (2018). Two's company, three's a crowd: Disabled people, their careers and their partners. *Disability & Society*, *33*(2), 272–284. https://doi.org/10.1080/09687599.2017.1399106

Milligan, M. S., & Neufeldt, A. H. (2001). The myth of asexuality: A survey of social and empirical evidence. *Sexuality and Disability*, *19*(2), 91–109. https://doi.org/10.1023/A:1010621705591

Molton, I. R., & Yorkston, K. M. (2017). Growing older with a physical disability: A special application of the successful aging paradigm. *The Journals of Gerontology: Series B, Psychological Sciences and Social Sciences*, *72*(2), 290–299. https://doi.org/10.1093/geronb/gbw122

Mudge, S., Rosie, J., Stott, S., Taylor, D., Signal, N., & McPherson, K. (2016). Ageing with cerebral palsy; What are the health experiences of adults with cerebral palsy? A qualitative study. *BMJ Open*, *6*(10), e012551. https://doi.org/10.1136/bmjopen-2016-012551

O'Dea, Z. (2018). The ayes have it! *The Qualitative Report*, *23*(10), 2313–2336. https://doi.org/10.46743/2160-3715/2018.2897

Paterson, L., McKenzie, K., & Lindsay, B. (2012). Stigma, social comparison and self-esteem in adults with an intellectual disability. *Journal of Applied Research in Intellectual Disabilities*, *25*(2), 166–176. https://doi.org/10.1111/j.1468-3148.2011.00651.x

Rainey, S. S. (2011). Love, sex, and disability: The pleasures of care. Boulder, CO: Lynne Rienner Publishers.

Riley, C. A. (2005). *Disability and the media: Prescriptions for change*. Hanover: University Press of New England.

Schalk, S. (2016). Reevaluating the supercrip. *Journal of Literary & Cultural Disability Studies*, *10*(1), 71–86, 128. https://doi.org/10.3828/jlcds.2016.5

Silverman, A. M., Molton, I. R., Smith, A. E., Jensen, M. P., & Cohen, G. L. (2017). Solace in solidarity: Disability friendship networks buffer well-being. *Rehabilitation Psychology*, *62*(4), 525–533. https://psycnet.apa.org/doi/10.1037/rep0000128

Vaccaro, A., Kimball, E., Newman, B. M., Moore, A., & Troiano, P. F. (2019). Collegiate purpose development at the intersections of disability and social class habitus. *Review of Higher Education*, *43*(1), 403–426. https://doi.org/10.1353/rhe.2019.0100

Watermeyer, B. (2017). I don't have time for an emotional life: Marginalization, dependency and melancholic suspension in disability. *Culture, Medicine and Psychiatry*, *41*(1), 142–160. https://doi.org/10.1007/s11013-016-9503-x

Wendell, S. (1996). *The rejected body: Feminist philosophical reflections on disability*. New York, NY: Routledge.

Westwood, S., & Carey, N. (2018). Ageing with physical disabilities and/or long-term health conditions. In S. Westwood (Ed.), *Ageing, diversity and equality: Social justice perspectives* (pp. 225–244). Routledge.

Young, S. (2014, June 9). *I'm not your inspiration, thank you very much* [Video]. TED Conferences. https://www.ted.com/talks/stella_young_i_m_not_your_inspiration_thank_you_very_much

Index

Note: Page numbers in *italic* refer to a figure on the corresponding page.

Made in the USA
Las Vegas, NV
19 September 2026

e5aac4ea-2d7a-4707-b800-838796f4e8a6R01